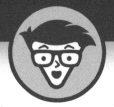

T0357586

Allergy

by **William E. Berger, MD, MBA**
Diplomate, American Board of Allergy & Immunology

Nicole M. Faris, MSc
Food Science & Technology
BSc Nutritional Science

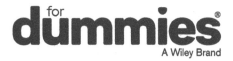

for **dummies**®
A Wiley Brand

Allergy For Dummies®

Published by: **John Wiley & Sons, Inc.**, 111 River Street, Hoboken, NJ 07030-5774, www.wiley.com

For general information on our other products and services, please contact our Customer Care Department within the U.S. at 877-762-2974, outside the U.S. at 317-572-3993, or fax 317-572-4002. For technical support, please visit https://hub.wiley.com/community/support/dummies.

Wiley publishes in a variety of print and electronic formats and by print-on-demand. Some material included with standard print versions of this book may not be included in e-books or in print-on-demand. For more information about Wiley products, visit www.wiley.com.

Library of Congress Control Number: 2024951718

ISBN: 978-1-394-25668-6 (pbk); ISBN 978-1-394-25670-9 (ebk); ISBN 978-1-394-25669-3 (ebk)

SKY10098489_021525

Allergy

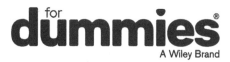

for
dummies®
A Wiley Brand

Contents at a Glance

Table of Contents

Introduction

"My nose won't stop running." "Oh, my aching sinuses." "I can't stop coughing." "My child keeps wheezing." If you've ever uttered words like these, you're not alone. These types of statements often describe allergies and/or asthma symptoms and are some of the most common medical complaints reported by people in the United States and around the world.

Allergens can cause a wide variety of medical conditions for millions of people all over the planet. These medical conditions can present as a minor annoyance, such as a runny nose; as a serious medical problem — for example, asthma; or even anaphylaxis, which is a potentially life-threatening reaction. Asthma itself affects more than 25 million people in the United States and is the most common chronic childhood disease and is now considered a global epidemic. And, according to the American Academy of Allergy, Asthma and Immunology, *allergic rhinitis* (hay fever) affects between 10 and 30 percent of the world's population. Food allergies are also increasing exponentially across the globe and have been reported to affect up to 8 percent of children and 10 percent of adults in the United States.

But enough about facts and figures. We want to talk about you: How are you feeling? Do you (or someone you know) think that feeling unwell is normal just because you have allergies and/or asthma and that the condition can never improve? Unfortunately, many people answer "yes" to this question. However, as we explain throughout this book, the plain, simple, and accurate medical truth is this: When you receive effective, appropriate care from your physician and you're a motivated participant in managing your allergic condition, you can lead a normal, active, and fulfilling life.

About This Book

We wrote this book to give you sound, up-to-date, practical advice — based on our more than 70 years of combined experience with numerous patients — about dealing with allergies and asthma effectively and appropriately. For that reason, the book is structured so that you can jump to sections that most directly apply to your medical condition. You don't need to read this book from cover to cover, although we won't object if you do. (Be careful, though, because when you start reading, you may have a really hard time putting it down!)

This book can also serve as a reference and source of information about the many facets of diagnosing, treating, and managing allergies and asthma. Although you may pick up this book to find out more about one aspect of allergies and asthma, you may realize later that other topics also apply to you or a loved one.

Don't worry about remembering where related subjects are in the book. We provide ample cross-references in every chapter that remind you where to look for the information you may need within other sections of the chapter you're currently reading or in other chapters.

The information in this book is designed to empower you as a person with allergies and/or asthma, thus helping you

>> Set goals for your treatment

>> Ensure that you receive the most appropriate and effective medical care for your allergic condition

>> Do your part as a patient by adhering to the treatment plan that you and your physician develop

Foolish Assumptions

We don't think it's too foolish to assume that you want substantive, scientifically accurate, relevant information about allergies and asthma, presented in everyday language, without a lot of medical mumbo jumbo. In this book, you find straightforward explanations of important scientific aspects of allergies and asthma and key medical terms. (You also get a chance to work on your Latin and Greek.)

If you've chosen to read our book, we know you're no dummy, so we're willing to go out on a limb and make some further assumptions about you, dear reader:

>> You or someone you care about suffers from allergies.

>> You want to find out more about allergies and asthma as part of improving your medical condition (in consultation with your physician, of course).

>> You want to feel better.

>> You really like physicians named Bill.

Icons Used in This Book

You may notice the following icons throughout the margins of the book. They're intended to catch your attention and alert you to the type of information presented in particular paragraphs. Here's what they mean:

DOCTOR SAYS

This icon represents Dr. Berger expressing his opinion.

REMEMBER

The Remember icon indicates things you shouldn't forget because you may find the information useful in the future.

SEE YOUR DOCTOR

The See Your Doctor icon alerts you to matters that you should discuss with your physician.

TECHNICAL STUFF

To give you as complete a picture as possible, we occasionally get into more complex details of medical science. The Technical Stuff icon lets you know that's what we're doing so you can delve into the topic further — or skip it. You don't have to read these paragraphs to understand the subject at hand. (However, reading the information with these icons may give you a better handle on managing your medical condition, as well as provide some great material for impressing your friends at your next party.)

TIP

You can find plenty of helpful information and advice in paragraphs marked with the Tip icon.

WARNING

A Warning icon advises you about potential problems, such as symptoms you shouldn't ignore or treatments you may not want to undergo.

Beyond This Book

The online Cheat Sheet at www.dummies.com provides an important list of myths and misconceptions about asthma and allergies, as well as a list of organs that are affected by allergy and asthma patients. We also include a Top Ten List of Common Allergy Triggers. Just search for "Allergy For Dummies Cheat Sheet" for this additional resource you can refer to whenever you need it.

Where to Go from Here

Although you can read this book from cover to cover if you want, we suggest turning to the table of contents and finding the sections that apply to your immediate concern. Then begin reading your way to better management of your allergies. Or you can search the index, find a topic that piques your interest, flip to that chapter, and read to your heart's content.

1

Getting Started with Allergy Basics

Understand allergic conditions and how they affect your overall health.

Diagnose and treat allergic disorders to improve your quality of life.

Recognize your immune system so you can better understand your allergic condition and work effectively with your physician.

Choose an allergist who can help treat your allergic symptoms and develop a shared decision plan together.

Know what to expect when you see your physician, including the types of examinations, procedures, and treatments that might be prescribed.

IN THIS CHAPTER

» **Introducing allergic ailments**

» **Connecting allergies and other conditions**

» **Defining the spectrum of allergic conditions**

» **Making sense of allergy signs and symptoms**

» **Recognizing life-threatening reactions**

Chapter **1**

Knowing What's Ailing You

llergy is a descriptive term for a wide variety of hypersensitivity disorders (meaning that you're excessively sensitive to one or more substances to which most people do not normally react).

Living a healthy, fulfilling life with allergies involves many of the same general diagnostic, treatment, and preventive measures that we explain throughout this book. In fact, the symptoms of seemingly disparate ailments such as *allergic rhinitis* (hay fever), most cases of asthma, *atopic dermatitis* (allergic eczema), food allergies, and other allergic conditions basically result from your immune system's similar, hyperreactive response to otherwise harmless substances that doctors refer to as *allergens*. This chapter serves as your entry point into the world of allergies.

Understanding How Allergies Cause Clinical Symptoms

The word *allergy* is the ancient Greek terms for an abnormal response or overreaction. Contrary to popular belief, weak or deficient immune systems don't cause asthma or allergy ailments. Rather, your body's defenses work overtime, making your immune system too sensitive to substances that pose a real threat to your well-being. That's why physicians often use the term *hypersensitivity* to refer to an allergy.

REMEMBER

These are the main points to keep in mind when dealing with allergies:

>> Allergies aren't just hay fever. In addition to affecting your nose, sinuses, eyes, and throat (as in typical cases of allergic rhinitis), exposure to allergy triggers can also cause symptoms that involve other organs of your body, including your lungs, skin, and digestive tract. Figure 1-1 shows all the organs in your body that allergies and asthma can affect.

>> These ailments aren't infections or contagious. You don't catch an allergy. However, as we explain in the section "Sensitizing your immune system" later in this chapter, you may inherit a genetic predisposition to develop hypersensitivities that can eventually appear as allergies.

>> Allergies aren't like trends or shoe sizes. You don't really outgrow them. Extensive studies in recent years show that although your ailment can certainly vary in character and severity over your lifetime, it's an ongoing physical condition that's most likely always present in some form.

>> Allergy triggers include allergens such as pollens, animal dander, dust mites, mold spores, various contact allergens, and certain foods, drugs, and venom from stinging insects. (See the section "Sensitizing your immune system" later in this chapter for more detailed classifications of these items.)

>> Clinical reactions can also result from nonallergic triggers that act as irritants, including tobacco smoke, household cleaners, aerosol products, solvents, chemicals, fumes, gases, paints, smoke, and indoor and outdoor air pollution.

>> Other forms of nonallergic triggers that can be mistaken as allergies are known as *precipitating factors* and include other medical conditions such as rhinitis, sinusitis, gastroesophageal reflux (GERD), and viral infections (colds, flu, COVID); physical stimuli such as exercise or variations in both air temperature and humidity levels; and sensitivities to food additives, such as sulfites, drugs such as beta-blockers (Inderal, Lopressor, Corgard, Timoptic), and aspirin and related over-the-counter nonsteroidal anti-inflammatory drugs (NSAIDs) such as ibuprofen (Advil, Motrin), ketoprofen (Actron, Orudis),

naproxen (Aleve), and newer prescription NSAIDs known as COX-2 inhibitors, such as celecoxib (Celebrex).

>> Allergies aren't mutually exclusive conditions. Having one type of hypersensitivity doesn't prevent you from developing others. You can have multiple sensitivities to different types of allergens, irritants, and precipitating factors. Many researchers (including Dr. Berger) consider allergic disorders a continuum of disease that can appear in many ways, depending on the nature and degree of your sensitivities, as well as your levels of exposure to triggers.

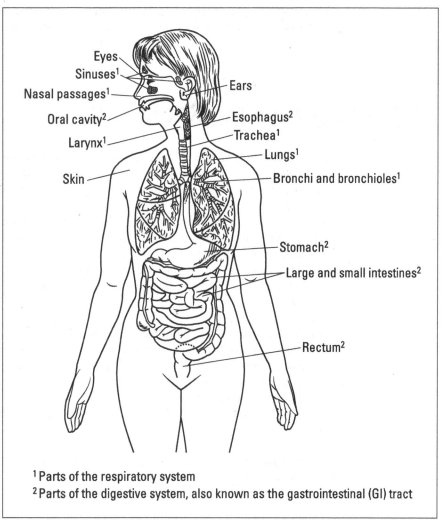

[1] Parts of the respiratory system
[2] Parts of the digestive system, also known as the gastrointestinal (GI) tract

FIGURE 1-1:
Allergies can affect organs throughout your body.

REMEMBER

>> All that sneezes, drips, runs, congests, wheezes, waters, coughs, itches, erupts, or swells isn't always due to an allergic reaction. That's why, as we explain in the section "Diagnosing and Treating Your Allergies" later in this chapter, the first step to effectively treating the underlying cause of your symptoms is properly diagnosing your ailment.

>> Although the majority of people with asthma also have allergies (and allergic rhinitis in most cases), some manifestations of asthma seem to develop without an allergic component. In cases of adult-onset asthma, which often develops in people older than 40 and is less common that child-onset asthma, *atopy* (a genetic tendency toward developing allergic hypersensitivity; see the next section) doesn't appear to play an important role. Instead, precipitating factors such as sinusitis, GERD, nasal polyps, and sensitivities to aspirin and related NSAIDs are more likely to trigger this condition.

Triggering Allergic Reactions

Your immune system acts as your second line of defense against foreign substances. The main barrier against foreign substances is your largest organ — your skin. (Remember that for your next appearance on *Jeopardy! Masters*.)

Usually, your immune system protects you against infectious bacteria, viruses, parasites, and other harmful agents by producing antibodies that learn to recognize the invaders and subsequently fend them off without too much fuss. In fact, most of the time, as long as your immune system works well, you may not even know that this constant, ongoing process takes place to ensure your survival and good health.

However, with an allergic condition, your immune system overproduces antibodies against typically harmless or inoffensive substances such as pollens. *Atopy* (the genetic susceptibility that can predispose your immune system to develop hypersensitivities) is the inherited characteristic that usually determines why some people's immune systems overreact and mount full-scale assaults when exposed to allergens, while others can ignore or innocuously eliminate those substances.

Here we explain atopy in more detail and describe how your family history may influence your risk of developing an allergic condition.

ALL IN THE ATOPIC FAMILY

Your genetically determined allergic predisposition (atopy) may present itself through different allergic conditions and target organs. This predisposition and a family history of allergies are the strongest predictors that you may develop asthma and/or other allergic conditions such as *allergic rhinitis* (hay fever), *atopic dermatitis* (allergic eczema), and food or drug hypersensitivities.

For example, your Uncle Ed may have allergic rhinitis, your sister may suffer from recurrent sinus and ear infections, and Cousin Al may have a childhood history of atopic dermatitis. Some of your especially unlucky relatives may even be "blessed" with a combination of all these allergic conditions, plus asthma, over the course of their lifetimes. (If you want to be the most popular member of your family, buy them a copy of this book.)

A typical atopic family history could consist of a person having atopic dermatitis as an infant, developing common atopic complications such as *otitis media* (ear infections — see Chapter 7) as a toddler, experiencing noticeable symptoms of allergic rhinitis in later childhood, and then developing asthma as a teenager.

However, an atopic history doesn't appear to put you at greater risk than the general population for developing allergic contact dermatitis (see Chapter 12) or allergic reactions to insect stings (see Chapter 17). These conditions seem affect nonallergic and allergic people alike, for reasons that we explain in Chapter 2.

Sensitizing your immune system

A complex sensitization process, in which your immune system responds to allergens, causes allergic reactions. Allergens that your immune system may respond to include the following:

>> Dust mites (see Chapter 4).

>> Pollens from certain grasses, weeds, and trees (see Chapter 4).

>> Mold spores (see Chapter 4).

>> Dander from many animals, including cats, dogs, rabbits, birds, horses, as well as gerbils, guinea pigs, and other pet rodents (see Chapter 5).

>> Foods, including peanuts, sesame, fish, shellfish, and tree nuts (in adults) and milk, eggs, soy and wheat (primarily in children). See Chapter 15 for more details.

>> The venom of stinging insects, including honeybees, wasps, yellow jackets, hornets, and fire ants, all of which belong to the *Hymenoptera* order of insects (see Chapter 17).

>> Drugs, including penicillin, and cephalosporins (see Chapter 16).

>> Contact allergens (see Chapter 12) such as poison ivy, oak, and sumac, as well as allergenic substances such as latex, nickel, and formaldehyde, which you can find in many everyday items. (See the section "Allergic contact dermatitis: Touching experiences" later in this chapter.)

Developing an allergic reaction

If you're predisposed to developing allergies, here's how a typical sensitization process and allergic reaction can develop, using ragweed pollen, one of the most common triggers of allergic rhinitis, as an example (you can find more details about this process in Chapter 2):

1. Ragweed pollen enters your body, usually as a result of inhaling it through your nose.

2. Your immune system detects the presence of these foreign substances in your body and stimulates the production of *IgE antibodies*, a special class of antibodies.

3. IgE antibodies attach themselves to the surfaces of mast cells that line tissues throughout your body, especially in your nose, eyes, lungs, and skin.

4. Your body designs IgE antibodies to counters specific substances.

   Your immune system is a magnificent memory machine: Unlike you or me, it hardly ever forgets a face. After sensitization occurs, you'll likely experience allergies to that substance for most of your life. With ragweed, for example, your immune system produces specific IgE antibodies with receptor sites that allow ragweed allergens to cross-link to the IgE ragweed-specific antibodies. The IgE antibodies work like a lock on the mast cell surface, and the allergen is the key. When the ragweed allergen connects with the two IgE antibodies on the mast cell surface, the bridging or docking mechanism unlocks the mast cell.

5. Unlocking the mast cell initiates the secretion of pro-inflammatory mediators such as histamines, leukotrienes, and other potent chemicals as a defensive response to the allergen.

   In turn, the actions of these chemicals trigger the swelling and inflammation that result in familiar allergy symptoms.

Physicians frequently use antihistamines to relieve allergy symptoms because histamine plays such an important role in the inflammatory process. There are now more specialized drugs to counter and/or inhibit some of the more fundamental allergic processes. In particular, inhaled corticosteroids, mast cell stabilizers, leukotriene modifiers, and new biologic monoclonal antibodies provide new therapeutic approaches to preventing and controlling symptoms of allergic and asthmatic reactions.

Managing Allergic Disease Effectively

In most parts of the world, allergies cause a wide range of problems for millions of people. Allergy problems can involve occasional minor symptoms, serious episodes and attacks, and even potentially life-threatening reactions (in the most severe cases).

However, thanks to recent medical breakthroughs in our understanding of the underlying allergic and immunological factors involved in allergic reaction, it's now possible in most cases to properly diagnose what's ailing you and to develop an appropriate and effective treatment plan for controlling your symptoms and managing your condition.

Effectively managing allergic conditions — particularly asthma and allergic rhinitis — frequently requires dealing with an assortment of symptoms, treatments, and preventive measures, because allergies (as well as asthma) tend to be ailments with many faces. Think of a typical Chinese restaurant menu: You many need to order dishes from different columns in order to have a complete meal. See Chapter 6 for information on managing your condition.

Previewing Allergic Conditions

Consider this part of the chapter a preview of forthcoming reactions. In the following sections, we touch on the significant features of the most common allergic diseases and provide important details about distinguishing them from nonallergic conditions that are similar. We also include references to the chapters where we discuss these ailments in more extensive detail.

Allergic rhinitis: Running away with your nose

Frequently referred to as *hay fever*, allergic rhinitis is the most common allergic disease in the United States. As many as 45 million Americans or more suffer from some form of this allergy. Trademark symptoms of allergic rhinitis include runny nose with clear, watery discharge; stuffy nose, sneezing; postnasal drip; and scratchy nose, ears, palate, and throat. In addition, itchy and watery eyes, symptoms of *allergic conjunctivitis* (inflammation or swelling of the eye due to an allergic reaction) are often associated with allergic rhinitis. Infections of the middle ear (known as the *otitis media*) and of the sinuses (*sinusitis*) are frequent complications of allergic rhinitis.

In Part 2 we discuss the many forms of allergic and nonallergic rhinitis, and we also explain the ways physicians diagnose and treat these ailments (including allergic conjunctivitis). We also share important tips on avoiding triggers of various types of rhinitis, details on medications, and information on the complications of allergic rhinitis symptoms.

Asthma: Breathing and wheezing

The most fundamental definition of *asthma* is a chronic, inflammatory airway disease of the lungs that causes breathing problems. However, in practice, asthma has many faces and is often difficult to recognize and properly diagnose. As a result, even though currently available prescription medications offer effective ways of relieving, preventing, and controlling the symptoms and underlying *inflammation* (redness, swellings, congestion, and disruption of normal processes of the airways of your lungs) that characterize asthma, the disease continues to cause serious problems for many people worldwide.

REMEMBER

Inflammation of the airways (*bronchial tubes*) is the most important underlying factor in asthma. In the vast majority of cases, if you have asthma, your symptoms may come and go, but the underlying inflammation usually persists.

Asthma's characteristic symptoms are coughing, wheezing, shortness of breath, chest tightness, and productive coughs (coughs that produce mucus). Important symptoms of asthma in infancy and early childhood include wheezing, persistent coughing, and recurring or lingering chest colds. (Because of its symptoms, asthma in children is often misdiagnosed as recurring bronchitis, recurring chest colds, or lingering coughs.) Asthma — like most allergies — is a manifestation of atopy. In fact, many people with asthma also have allergic rhinitis.

The hyperreactive response of the sensitized immune system to asthmatic triggers (typically inhalant allergens, such as dander and dust mites, as well as other substances, including irritants, which also trigger allergic rhinitis symptoms) is usually the main factor in aggravating the underlying airway inflammation (see Chapter 8 for a detailed explanation of this process).

In Part 3 we examine asthma, including diagnosis, treatment, ways to avoid asthma triggers, asthma medications, long-term asthma management, and special considerations involving asthma during pregnancy and childhood.

Atopic dermatitis: Scratching your itch

Also describes as *atopic eczema* or *allergic eczema*, atopic dermatitis is an allergic condition that targets your body's largest organ — your skin. The simplest way to define this noncontagious skin condition is the itch that scratches (or the "itch that rashes").

REMEMBER

"The itch that scratches" refers to the itch-scratch cycle, the hallmark of atopic dermatitis. Scratching your dry skin causes more irritation and inflammation, further damaging your skin and making it even itchier, resulting in more scratching and increasingly irritated skin. Eventually, fissures and cracks can develop on your skin, allowing irritants, bacteria, and viruses to enter, often leading to complicating infections.

Atopic dermatitis frequently occurs with allergic rhinitis and can also precede other allergic symptoms. As such, atopic dermatitis can provide an early clue that you're at risk of developing other allergies and asthma.

This section just scratches the surface of information on atopic dermatitis. If you're itching for more, see Chapter 11.

IT'S IN YOUR AIRWAYS, NOT IN YOUR HEAD

For centuries, many people believed that psychological factors such as anxiety, emotional disorders, or stress cause asthma. However, although these problems can *aggravate* asthma or allergies, they don't by themselves *cause* asthma or allergies.

Unfortunately, we still hear about the friends and family of people with asthma who claim that asthma is all in the patient's head. Some of these people insist that if the person would just calm down, their condition would go away. Instead of stress causing asthma, it can be the other way around: Breathing problems can cause stress. Stressing out because you can't breathe is a perfectly normal and understandable response.

(continued)

(continued)

Therefore, a proper diagnosis of asthma and/or allergies, and early, aggressive treatment for these conditions are crucial. In most cases, you should be able to control your asthma and allergic condition so that it doesn't control you, thus enabling you to lead a full and active life. Forget the negative stereotypes of people with asthma and people with allergies as nerdy, weak, anxious types, forever coughing and blowing their noses. Asthma and allergies can affect anyone: from the captain of the school chess team to the captain of the football team, as well as everybody in between.

Allergic contact dermatitis: Touching experiences

Although you may not know it, you're probably already familiar with allergic contact dermatitis, because one of the most common triggers of this condition is poison ivy and other related plants of the *Toxicodendron* family. Other important triggers include latex, nickel, and formaldehyde.

REMEMBER

The characteristic signs of allergic contact dermatitis include red rash, swollen pimples, blisters, and itchy skin. These symptoms may appear hours to days after your skin contacts an allergen, and they usually develop where the allergen touches the skin. As you may expect, the point of allergen entry is where the skin usually shows the most severe inflammation. Chapter 12 provides more detailed information on diagnosing and treating allergic contact dermatitis, avoiding triggers of this allergy, and preventing poison ivy from ruining your picnic or camping trip.

Urticaria and angioedema: Breaking out and swelling up

Urticaria and *angioedema*, better known as hives and deep swelling, can present perplexing problems. Figuring out why hives happen could give you hives — if that weren't one of the most common misconceptions about these skin eruptions. In fact, contrary to popular belief, stress and other psychological factors aren't the primary causes of hives but may possibly aggravate a pre-existing condition.

REMEMBER

Another common myth is that hives and *angioedema* (deep swellings) always result from allergic reactions. In fact, although allergies can cause some cases of *acute* (rapid onset) hives and angioedema, more often these eruptions occur as a result of nonallergic mechanisms, especially in cases of chronic hives.

Angioedema usually coexists with hives. Deep swellings that develop without hives can indicate a serious underlying disorder or may signal a severe, adverse drug reaction.

REMEMBER

The most common allergic triggers of hives and angioedema are

>> Food hypersensitivities, especially peanuts, tree nuts, milk, eggs, fish, shellfish, soybean, sesame, and fruits such as melons and berries. (See Chapter 14 for more information on food allergies.)

>> Insect stings from insects of the *Hymenoptera* order (honeybees, yellow jackets, wasps, hornets, and fire ants) can often cause small, localized hives that develop into blisters if you're sensitized to the venom of these insects. In rare cases, *anaphylaxis*, a life-threatening reaction that affects many organs simultaneously (see the section "Anaphylaxis: Severe systemic symptoms" later in this chapter), can follow an insect sting. Refer to Chapter 17 for more information on insect stings.

>> Medications, including penicillin, sulfa drugs, and other antibiotics; aspirin and nonsteroidal anti-inflammatory drugs (NSAIDs); insulin; narcotic pain relievers; muscle relaxants; and tranquilizers can trigger systemic hives if you have sensitivities to allergens in these products. See Chapter 16 for more information on drug reactions. Chapter 13 goes into much deeper detail about hives and angioedema.

Food hypersensitivities: Serving up allergens

Most adverse food reactions aren't the result of true *food hypersensitivities* (the more precise terms for food allergies). In fact, various forms of food intolerance, food poisoning, and other nonallergic mechanisms cause the majority of reactions that most people blame on food allergies.

REMEMBER

The most frequent triggers of actual food hypersensitivities are proteins in the following foods:

>> Peanuts and other legumes, including soybeans, peas, lentils, beans, and foods containing these ingredients

>> Shellfish, including crustaceans and mollusks such as shrimp, lobster, crab, clams, mussels, and oysters

>> Fish, both freshwater and saltwater

- » Tree nuts, including almonds, Brazil nuts, cashews, hazelnuts, pistachios, pecans, and walnuts

- » Eggs, especially egg whites

- » Cow's milk, including products that contain casein and whey

- » Soy, including soy products like soy milk, tofu, tempeh, and miso.

- » Wheat and other grains and cereals, such as corn, rice, barley, and oats

- » Sesame from foods that contain sesame seeds, such as hummus

SEE YOUR DOCTOR

In cases in which mouth and lip swelling, wheezing, or hives occur immediately after consuming a particular food (peanuts, for example), you many easily deduce that an allergic response caused your reaction. However, in many other instances, distinguishing between food intolerance and true food hypersensitivity can require more extensive diagnostic procedures. If you're hungry for more information on adverse food reactions, see Chapter 15.

Drug hypersensitivities: Taking the wrong medicine

Certain drugs are prone to produce allergic reactions in susceptible individuals. The most frequent type of adverse allergic reactions to medications occurs with penicillin and its related compounds. Aspirin and related NSAIDs — including newer prescription NSAIDs, known as COX-2 inhibitors, such as celecoxib (Celebrex) — and other drugs can also trigger adverse reactions. However, most adverse drug reactions result from nonallergic mechanisms, as we discuss in Chapter 16.

Although drug hypersensitivity reactions most frequently target the skin, adverse allergic reactions to drugs can affect any organ system in your body, including mucous membranes, lymph nodes, kidneys, liver, lungs, and joints. These reactions can trigger skin rashes, hives, angioedema, respiratory symptoms such as coughing or wheezing, fever (sometimes resulting in drug fever, occasionally with shaking chills and a skin rash), and low blood pressure and /or anemia, resulting from an adverse reaction that destroys your red blood cells.

WARNING

In less frequent but more serious cases, an adverse drug reaction can result in anaphylaxis, a severe, potentially life-threatening response that affects many organs simultaneously (see the section "Anaphylaxis: Severe systemic symptoms" later in this chapter). In fact, penicillin injections cause the most drug-related anaphylactic deaths in the United States. (Fortunately, the use of penicillin shots has significantly decreased in recent years.) For more information on drug hypersensitivities, see Chapter 16.

Stinging insects: The wrong kind of buzz

The venom of stinging insects from the *Hymenoptera* order (honeybees, yellow jackets, wasps, hornets, and fire ants) can trigger allergic reactions in people who are sensitized to those allergens. Reactions range from discomfort, swelling, itching, and hives to — in rare cases — potentially life-threatening anaphylaxis.

Like allergic contact dermatitis, insect-sting hypersensitivities are equal-opportunity allergies. Having other allergic conditions, such as allergic rhinitis, asthma, atopic dermatitis, or food allergies, or a family history of atopy puts you at no greater risk than anyone else for experiencing an allergic reaction to stings from these insects.

In Chapter 17, we provide extensive details on these insects and how you can avoid venomous encounters with them.

Anaphylaxis: Severe systemic symptoms

WARNING

Anaphylaxis, an ultimate but thankfully rare form of allergic reaction, involves a severe, potentially life-threatening response that affects many organs simultaneously. The characteristic signs of anaphylaxis include

>> Flushing (sudden reddening of the skin)

>> Dramatic itching over the entire body

>> Itchy rash or hives

>> Nausea, vomiting, abdominal pain, and/or diarrhea

>> Swelling of the throat and/or tongue (limbs may also swell)

>> Difficulty breathing

>> Dizziness or fainting

>> Severe drop in blood pressure

REMEMBER

The most frequent causes of anaphylaxis in the United States are extreme allergic reactions to the following allergens:

>> Venom from stinging insects of the *Hymenoptera* order

>> Drugs such as penicillin and related compounds

>> Foods — particularly peanuts and shellfish

In addition, *pseudoallergic* or *idiosyncratic reactions* (see Chapter 16) caused by drugs such as aspirin or related OTC NSAIDs like ibuprofen (Advil, Motrin), ketoprofen (Actron, Orudis), naproxen (Aleve), and newer prescription NSAIDs, known as COX-2 inhibitors, including celecoxib (Celebrex), can (in some cases) lead to severe, potentially life-threatening reactions referred to as a non IgE-mediated immune response or as an *anaphylactoid reaction*, involving direct activation of certain immune cells such as mast cells and basophils (see Chapter 2).

If you're at risk of anaphylaxis, you should be prepared to take emergency measures to prevent this type of extremely serious reaction. Consult with your physician about prescribing an emergency kit (such as EpiPen or Auvi-Q) that contains an injectable dose of epinephrine, or the single dose epinephrine nasal spray called "neffy," which was recently approved by the U.S. Food and Drug Administration (FDA).

TIP

Make sure that your physician shows you how to use the injectable device. Learning the proper technique for administering epinephrine in your physician's office is much more effective than trying it out for the first time while you're having a reaction.

Because anaphylaxis is such a serious issue and can result from various types of exposures, we address it throughout the book, wherever applicable.

DYEING YOUR ALLERGIES

Inhaled topical corticosteroids, which are often used as asthma and allergy treatments — including budesonide (Pulmicort, Rhinocort), mometasone (Asmanex, Nasonex), and other inhaled topical corticosteroid products that we list in Chapter 6 — are extremely effective in suppressing the inflammatory process. Keep in mind, however, that most asthma and allergy drugs treat the end result of a long, complex chain of immune system reactions but don't fundamentally prevent the underlying process causing your ailment. Therefore, if you stop taking your prescribed medications, the underlying disease process most likely restarts, and your clinical symptoms reappear.

We compare this process to dyeing your hair. You can change your hair color, but if you don't continue coloring it (like treating your asthma and allergies with your prescribed medicine), your new hair growth comes in with its original color, because you haven't really altered its underlying, genetically determined characteristics.

Diagnosing and Treating Allergic Disorders: Just the Basics

The basic components of effectively managing allergies include the following steps.

» **Getting a proper diagnosis of your condition**. Identifying the specific allergens, irritants, and/or precipitating factors that may trigger your ailment is a critical component of your diagnosis. Cough medicine isn't the treatment for your cough if you have asthma. First finding out why you're coughing (cough may be the only obvious symptom of underlying asthma in certain patients) is vital so you can then take appropriate steps to effectively control and manage your condition.

» **Avoiding or reducing exposures to allergens, irritants, and precipitating factors that may trigger your asthma and/or allergies.** Effective avoidance and allergy-proofing measures (see Chapters 5 and 9) can significantly improve your quality of life and often reduce, or in certain cases eliminate, your need for medication.

» **Taking long-term preventive medications to control your underlying condition while appropriately using short-term medications when you experience flare-ups, episodes, or attacks.** We provide extensive information on prescription and over-the-counter allergy and asthma products in Chapters 6 and 10.

» **Evaluating and monitoring your condition.** Consider having a comprehensive evaluation by a board-certified allergist to confirm your diagnosis and to follow your clinical course.

» **Adhering to your treatment plan and keeping yourself informed about all aspects of your condition.** Follow the recommendation of your physician, take your medicines as prescribed, and come prepared with any questions you might have at the time of your office appointments.

» **Keeping yourself in good general health (by eating healthy and exercising) to avoid developing more severe symptoms or potential complications of your ailment and to help you enjoy the highest quality of life possible.** Good health and an active lifestyle will certainly help you maintain an excellent quality of life and allow you to participate in the activities that bring you enjoyment.

CLIMATE CHANGE AND THE INCREASING INCIDENCE OF ALLERGIC CONDITIONS

A significant factor contributing to the increase in allergic disorders in recent years, is climate change. Warmer temperatures coupled with increased carbon dioxide levels in the atmosphere, create ideal conditions for plants to produce more pollen, lengthening seasonal allergies and intensifying pollen concentrations.

This prolonged exposure to allergens exacerbates existing allergies and may even trigger new allergies in sensitive individuals. The extreme weather events, caused by climate change, such as intense heatwaves and flooding, worsen air quality by increasing environmental pollutants and mold spores, which further aggravates respiratory allergies such as asthma and allergic rhinitis.

Chapter **2**

Understanding Your Immune System

I n terms of germs, the world can still be a rough place. Despite major advances during the last 100 years in fighting infectious diseases and providing effective medical care for increasing numbers of people, viruses, bacteria, fungi, and other potentially harmful agents remain constant threats to your health. That's why your body's defense network is so important to your well-being.

Your front-line defense against potentially infections intruders is the physical barrier formed by your body's largest organ — your skin. (Your mucus membranes, as well as the highly acidic digestive juices of your stomach, the beneficial bacteria in your gut, and certain nonspecific cells, also act as immediate defenders against uninvited guests.) The second far more complex and fundamental defense apparatus in your body — and one of the most important keys to the survival of the human species — is your immune system.

Because numerous immune system processes can play important roles as underlying factors in allergy and asthma (as well as in many other diseases), doctors frequently need to apply their understanding of *immunology* (the science of immunity) when evaluating and treating allergic conditions.

We devote this chapter to explaining the immunologic basis of allergic reactions so that you can have a better understanding of what may be at the root of your ailment and to review with you what your physician considers when diagnosing and treating your condition.

Protecting Your Health: How Your Immune System Works

The most basic function of your immune system is to distinguish between your body (self) and potentially harmful (non-self) agents. Your immune system performs the following functions to protect you:

>> Recognizes foreign (therefore, potentially harmful) microorganisms, their products, and toxins, all known generally as *antigens*. These substances can stimulate a response from your immune system and react with an antibody or a sensitized *T-cell* (a specialized immune system cell involved in cell-mediated immunity, as we explain in "Reacting to allergen exposures," later in this chapter). Allergens, which usually consist of proteins, are particular types of antigens, which initiate an allergic response.

>> Identifies self-antigens. These antigens are usually damaged and/or improperly functioning cells in your body. Malignant cells that can develop into tumor-causing cancerous cells are an example of self-antigens.

>> Assists in removing antigens from your body.

The immune system defense is vital to the survival of all animals. If your immune system functions properly, its protective function is an underlying, ongoing, and generally imperceptible aspect of your everyday existence.

TECHNICAL STUFF

Your immune system can work as a double-edged sword, however. In some cases, it deploys its defensive functions too zealously while trying to protect your body against any type of perceived threat. In such cases, rather than preventing infections, your immune system can actually instigate certain types of health problems, including

>> **Autoimmune disorders:** These disorders include serious diseases such as rheumatic fever, a rare complication of an inadequately treated strep infection of the upper respiratory tract (strep throat), in which the immune system can attack heart tissue cells that cross-react with *Streptococcus* bacterial antigens. This kind of complication is why it's so important that you take the full course of antibiotic therapy your physician prescribes for strep throat and that you return to your doctor's office of a repeat throat culture to

make sure that your infection has completely resolved. (For more information on cross-reactivity, see Chapter 5.)

In other cases, the immune system (for reason researchers are still trying to discover) loses its ability to distinguish between certain self and non-self substances. This inability to make that distinction can cause diseases such as systemic lupus erythematous, psoriasis, rheumatoid arthritis, and some forms of diabetes, when your immune system perceives otherwise functional and vital cells in your body as antigens and turns its firepower on them.

>> **Rejection of organ transplants:** Doctors usually try to find a close genetic match between patient and organ donors to reduce the risk of the patient's immune system rejecting the donated organ. In many cases, however, physicians still need to administer drugs to suppress the patient's immune system and prevent organ rejection. This suppression of the immune system can then increase the risk of opportunistic infections potentially harming the patient.

>> **Allergic conditions:** If you have allergies or asthma, you almost certainly have an immune system that works too well or overreacts. As we explain in Chapter 1, doctors use the term *hypersensitivity* to refer to allergies because your immune system is overly sensitive to substances such as certain food proteins, carbohydrates, pollens, animal dander, and other types of allergens that offer no real threat to your health. With hypersensitivity, your immune system acts like an alarm system that summons a SWAT team regardless of whether a cat burglar or just a cat is intruding on your property.

Classifying Immune System Components and Disorders

Your immune system consists of several related processes. Think of these processes as a civil defense network of arsenals, supply lines, logistical support, and command and control centers for the cells that actually defend your body. The most important organ and tissue components of your immune system include the following:

>> **Bone marrow:** This is where stem cells (early, non-specific types of cells) originate, developing into *B-cells* (specialized types of plasma cells) that subsequently secrete distinct forms of plasma proteins, known as *antibodies*. These antibodies are divided into the following five classes of *immunoglobulins* (identified by the prefix Ig):

- **IgG:** The major component of gammaglobulin used for treating certain types of immune deficiencies, IgG antibodies account for at least three-quarters of the antibodies in your body. This class of antibodies, together with IgM antibodies, in cooperation with your white blood cells, is vital in defending you against bacterial infections. IgG antibodies also play an important role in preventing allergens from initiating an allergic reaction. As a response to *immunotherapy* (allergy shots), the production of IgG antibodies is believed to work by blocking IgE antibodies from binding to mast cells, thus preventing the subsequent release of chemical mediators of inflammation that produce allergy and asthma symptoms. (See "Reacting to allergen exposures," later in this chapter for more information.)

- **IgM:** About 5 percent of your antibodies belong to this class, which plays a role in the primary immune response and also enhances the role of IgG antibodies.

- **IgA:** The primary antibody in your mucus membrane surfaces, IgA antibodies reside in your saliva, tears, and in the secretions of the mucosal surfaces of your respiratory bronchi, gastrointestinal, and genital tracts, where these antibodies protect against infection. They're also present in mother's milk for the first few days after giving birth, thus providing antibody protection (referred to as *passive immunity*) for breast-fed newborns.

- **IgD:** This antibody class, which works with the antigen at cell surface contact, seems to exist in very small quantities and plays a nonspecific role in the immune process.

- **IgE:** Although present in only minute quantities in your body, IgE antibodies (also known as *reaginic antibodies)* are key players in allergic reactions (hence the longer paragraphs; these antibodies are probably the reason you're reading this book). Although everyone produces IgE antibodies, allergy sufferers have an inherited tendency to overproduce these agents. IgE antibodies can induce other cells, particularly mast cells and basophils (special sentinel cells, as we explain in "Reacting to allergen exposures," later in this chapter), to set in motion a complex chain reaction that culminates in your allergy and asthma symptoms.

  Mast cell surfaces have special IgE receptor sites. Two allergen-specific IGE antibodies linking to an allergen (such as pollen, animal dander, molds, dust mite allergens, insect sting venom, and certain foods and drugs) on the surface of the mast cell can trigger a Type 1 allergic reaction, also known as an IgE mediated allergic reaction (see "Classifying Abnormal Immune Responses," later in this chapter).

>> **Cytokines:** These signaling proteins play an important role in nearly all aspects of inflammation and immunity. They're chemical messengers that tell your cells how to behave. Some cytokines make disease worse (proinflammatory), while others act to reduce inflammation and have a healing effect (anti-inflammatory). *Interleukins* are a group of cytokines that act as chemical signals between white blood cells. The major anti-inflammatory cytokines include interleukin-4 (IL-4), IL-6, IL-10, IL-11, and IL-13. Inflammatory cytokines include interleukin-1 (IL-1), IL-12, and IL-18. Interleukin-5 (IL-5) is known to be a pro-inflammatory cytokine that controls the production, activation, and localization of eosinophils that mediate allergy and asthma symptoms.

>> **TSLP:** Thymic stromal lymphopoietin is an epithelial cell-derived cytokine expressed in the skin, gut, lungs, and thymus. It activates dendritic cells to promote T helper (Th) 2 immune reactions. It's a key mediator of asthma and can cause severe allergic airway inflammatory responses by its action on adaptive and innate immune cells and structural cells.

>> **Thymus:** Secretions of special hormones (such as thymosin) from this gland are vital for regulating your immune system's functions. The thymus also helps encode certain T-cells, which then play key role in developing antibodies against antigens.

>> **Lymph nodes:** The lymphatic system provides drainage for your immune system. Your lymph nodes filter out material resulting from a local inflammatory reaction. If you seem to have, for example, strep throat, your doctor checks for swollen lymph nodes downstream from the infected area (under your throat) as an indication of infection.

>> **Spleen:** This organ filters and processes antigens in your blood.

>> **Lymphoid tissues:** These important immune system participants, which include your tonsils, adenoids, appendix and parts of your intestines, help process antigens.

DOCTOR SAYS

INFLAMING YOU FOR A GOOD REASON

You may wonder why you're equipped with IgE antibodies if they're so problematic. This seemingly bothersome immunoglobulin is a significant part of the reason the human species made it to another millennium. During prehistoric times, in addition to the challenges of hunting and gathering our daily meal (and trying not to become another animal's chow in the process), humans also had to contend with all sorts of infectious agents, especially parasites.

(continued)

(continued)

The potent inflammatory action triggered when a parasite-specific antigen would bind with cell-bound IgE antibodies probably insured that parasitic infections couldn't affect enough humans to endanger our species. In fact, IgE antibodies remain important players in the immune responses of some people in less-developed regions of the world, where parasites continue to pose threats to human health. I have seen patients who have recently arrived from less-developed countries and who have highly elevated IgE and eosinophil levels in their blood tests. In those cases, I rule out parasitic infections before moving to a more likely diagnosis of an allergic condition. However, because parasites are such an extremely rare problem in the U.S. population, elevated IgE and eosinophil levels are almost always a sign that I'm dealing with an allergic patient.

In most modern-day humans, IgE antibodies play a role similar to that of fat cells. In prehistoric times, humans needed fat cells to store food and stave off hunger when their hunting and gathering was less than productive. Now, human fat cells turn into love handles, and IgE antibodies trigger allergies.

Protecting and serving in many ways

The protective mechanisms of your immune system consist of several basic components. Think of these components as separate armed forces branches that use different but related means to accomplish the immune system's overall defense mission. The six basic components are

>> **Humoral immunity:** This component (which is not a vaccine against stand-up comedians) acts similarly to an internal air force, using *B cells* (see "Classifying Immune System Components and Disorders") to produce and deploy antibodies (the immune system's equivalent of high-tech weaponry). This component provides your body with its primary defense mechanism against bacterial infection and also plays a major role in developing allergies in people with a family history of *atopy* (the genetic susceptibility that can predispose the immune system to develop hypersensitivities and produce antibodies to otherwise harmless allergens).

>> **Cell-mediated immunity:** This component uses *T cells* (see "Protecting Your Health: How Your Immune System Works" earlier in this chapter) and related cell products (sort of like the army, battling in the trenches), rather than antibodies, to directly protect you against viruses, fungi, intracellular organisms, and tumor antigens.

>> **Phagocytic immunity:** The function of this component is similar to a mop-up squad (or vultures and other scavengers), because it uses so-called

scavenger cells (macrophages) that circulate throughout your body, looking for debris to clean up. This form of immunity doesn't play a significant role in the allergic process.

>> **Complement:** This term describes a composite system of plasma and cell membrane proteins that interact with one another, as well as with antibodies, and serve as important mediators in your civil defense system, protecting the home front like the Coast Guard. Diseases associated with complement deficiency vary depending on which component of the complement system is lacking. Some people may have an increased susceptibility to infection, some may experience a rheumatic disorder (such as lupus erythematous or rheumatoid arthritis), and some may have hereditary angioedema (deep swellings) that occur without hives and can potentially cause life-threatening symptoms (see Chapter 13).

>> **Innate immunity:** Your body's innate immunity triggers an immune response to a harmful foreign substance or pathogen. This innate immunity is general and nonspecific and isn't dependent on antigen specific immunity. In other words, it's something already in the body that plays a protective role in keeping you healthy.

>> **Adaptive immunity:** Your body also has the capability of developing adaptive immunity in response to a foreign substance. This form of immunity is specific and responds only to certain types of infections or vaccinations. For example, if you've had measles or received a measles vaccine, you're protected against measles by your adaptive immune system for life, but not against other viruses such as polio or chicken pox. Therefore, it's vital for you and your child to receive all of the different types of recommended vaccines in order to stay healthy.

Distinguishing between immune deficiencies and allergic conditions

Years ago, when *immune deficiency* was mentioned, people needed an extensive explanation of the subject. Now healthcare professionals spend most of their time clarifying that immunodeficiency isn't synonymous with AIDS (Acquired Immunodeficiency Syndrome), but rather that AIDS represents just one out of a whole multitude of immune deficiency diseases.

REMEMBER

If your physician advises testing for immune deficiency, they aren't necessarily ordering an HIV test (which causes AIDS). Instead, your physician is most likely ordering immune deficiency tests to rule out other types of diseases.

Although allergy and asthma conditions are almost always synonymous with a hyperreactive immune system, rare cases exist in which people with IgA deficiencies, who have recurring infections, may also have allergic conditions. However, immune deficiencies of any type are very rare when compared to the overall incidence of allergies and asthma.

REMEMBER

Keep the following important points about immunodeficiencies and allergy and asthma in mind:

>> In most cases, if you have allergies and asthma and a history of recurring infections, your overresponsive immune system is actually swamping your system with excess mucus that gets infected and is indirectly causing your infections such as sinusitis (Chapter 7) or bronchitis (Chapter 9).

DOCTOR SAYS

>> In many decades of treating thousands of patients referred to me for recurring infections, I've seen only a handful of patients with immune deficiencies. In the vast majority of cases, I found that these patients had allergies and/or asthma.

>> If you have a bacterial infection such as acute sinusitis or bronchitis, your physician should evaluate whether your infection is a complication of allergic rhinitis and/or asthma before checking for much less common immune deficiencies.

WARNING

>> Doctors can rule out most immune deficiency syndromes by using simple blood tests that measure your blood count and antibody levels. For this reason, we strongly advise against indiscriminately receiving gammaglobulin therapy unless you first have an immune work-up that reveals a significant deficiency requiring this kind of treatment.

Immunizing and immunology

You often hear that life is a constant learning process. This statement is especially true for your immune system. In fact, your immune system is a seemingly limitless learning machine that constantly memorizes the characteristics of countless antigens in order to create memories of these encounters that allow your defenses to react to exposures in the future.

The memory chips of any computer that you or we are likely to use in our lifetimes pale in comparison to the virtual total recall of the immune system. Through the humoral component (see "Protecting and serving in many ways," earlier in this chapter). Your immune system can recognize hundreds of trillions of antigens and produce specific antibodies against each and every one of these substances. Compare this feat to remembering the name, looks, and characteristics of every single person, animal, and plant that you encounter throughout your lifetime (which could come in handy at your high school reunion).

Memorizing menaces to your health

Your immune system's phenomenal capacity to memorize explains how having a particular viral infection usually enables you to acquire immunity to that specific virus for the future. Your immune system usually recognizes the antigen on subsequent exposure, thus triggering a rapid response from its specialized mechanisms and cells, which neutralize and dispose of the offending virus before it can adversely affect you.

TECHNICAL
STUFF

Many ancient cultures recognized that people who survived infectious diseases were usually immunized against catching the same ailment again. In fact, ancient Chinese and Egyptian doctors practiced limited forms of immunization.

Fooling your immune system for your own good.

Immunization tricks your immune system into thinking that you've actually had a full-blown infection, without risking the potentially life-threatening consequences that a disease such as polio can cause. Your immune system's reaction to the perceived infection ensures that if you ever receive exposure to that same pathogen, your defensive mechanisms will respond rapidly and effectively, thus protecting your health.

Vaccines developed thanks to advances in immunology are the main reason that parents in the United States and many other parts of the world no longer need to worry about their children succumbing to a summer epidemic of polio. Other diseases that medical science has successfully brought under control as a result of immunizations include smallpox, diphtheria, pertussis (whopping cough), respiratory syncytial virus (RSV), tetanus, chicken pox, shingles, measles, German measles (rubella), and mumps, as well as forms of hepatitis and meningitis.

In fact, stimulating your immune system into producing a protective immune response against allergens is the underlying basis of immunotherapy, as we explain in the section "Reaping the Benefits of Immunology" later in this chapter.

Classifying Abnormal Immune Responses

Your immune system can cause you trouble when it malfunctions, either because of a deficiency or by doing its job too well. Scientists refer to these abnormal responses according to distinct classifications of reactions, which we discuss in the following sections.

REMEMBER

Although allergic responses can involve aspects of all five types of these mechanisms, Types I and IV, which process and memorize previous antigen encounters, are most important in the vast majority of allergic conditions.

IgE -mediated reactions (Type I)

IgE-mediated reactions (Type I) result in immediate allergic reactions. Also known as *immediate hypersensitivity,* they often result from an insect sting or the injection of a drug such as penicillin in people who have extreme sensitivities to these triggers. The most dramatic and dangerous Type I reaction is anaphylaxis (see Chapter 1).

Allergic rhinitis (hay fever), allergic asthma, food allergies, and certain types of skin and drug allergies are other examples of this type of immune mechanism. Because of the sudden onset of the allergic reaction in cases of immediate hypersensitivity, allergy skin testing (see Chapter 4) can provide quick results in identifying the triggers of those conditions in many cases. For a more in-depth explanation of Type I reactions, see "Developing an Immediate Hypersensitivity" later in this chapter.

Cytotoxic reactions (Type II)

Cytotoxic reactions (Type II) involve destruction of cells, such as the reactions that result in the breakdown of red blood cells. This mechanism can potentially lead to anemia and fewer platelets in the blood, a situation that decreases your blood's ability to clot.

Certain drugs such as penicillin, sulfonamides, and quinidine can trigger cytotoxic reactions. Type II reactions play a role in Rh-factor anemia and jaundice in newborns and are also the way a patient's body may reject an organ transplant.

Immune complex reactions (Type III)

Manifestations of *immune complex reactions (Type III)* include fever, skin rash, hives, swollen, tender lymph nodes, and aching or painful joints. These types of reactions are among the ones that physicians usually refer to as *serum sickness.* Typically, these symptoms appear one to three weeks after taking final doses of drugs such as penicillin, sulfonamides, thiouracil, and phenytoin. For example, in systemic lupus erythematosus, circulating immune complexes deposit on organs such as the kidneys, joints, skin, heart, and lungs.

Cell-mediated reactions (Type IV)

Allergic contact dermatitis is one of the primary examples of *cell-mediated reactions* (*Type IV*), a localized, nonsystemic reaction (Chapter 12). Doctors also use the term *delayed hypersensitivity* to describe this process, in which contact with an allergen results in an allergic reaction hours or even days later. (For example, if you have allergic contact dermatitis, you may not realize that you've contacted poison ivy until you're driving home from your weekend camping trip.)

Stimulatory hypersensitivity (Type V)

This type of reaction is one in which antibodies are made against a specific hormone receptor of a hormone–producing cell, stimulating specific cell targets. This causes an overstimulation of hormone producing cells. his reaction is seen in hyperthyroidism (Grave's disease) where antibodies that stimulate the thyroid-stimulating hormone receptor leads to overactivity or the thyroid gland.

Developing an Immediate Hypersensitivity

Type I allergic reactions involve numerous complex processes, with many players taking part in various ways. The following sections explain the roles that most important cells and chemicals play in developing your sensitivities and triggering your reactions and provide an overview to the sequence of events involved in sensitizing your immune system and triggering subsequent allergic reactions.

Setting the stage for allergic reactions

Significant cell participants in Type I reactions include the following:

>> **Mast cells:** These connective-tissue cells play a pivotal role in allergic disease processes. Mast cells are primarily located near blood vessel and mucus-producing cells in the tissues that line various parts of your body. With allergies and asthma, doctors concern themselves with your mast cells' actions in the lining of your eyes, ears, nose, sinuses, throat, the airways of your lungs, your skin, and even your gastrointestinal (GI) tract.

REMEMBER

>> **Basophils:** These cells live in your bloodstream near the surfaces of tissue and are important players in late-phase reactions. (See "Reacting to allergen exposures," later in this chapter for more information.)

Mast cells and basophils are among the first cells that antigens encounter when entering your body. These sentinel cells are coated with numerous IgE receptor sites that can bind IgE antibodies that are specific to various allergens (corresponding, for example, to different foods and pollens, dust mites, and animal danders).

These cells also contain potent chemical mediators of inflammation that are released when IgE and a specific allergen cross-link on the cell surface and activate them, resulting in the inflammation that leads to allergy and asthma symptoms.

>> **Eosinophils:** Other mediators, called *chemotactic factors*, attract these white blood cells to the site of an allergic reaction where they generate an array of other inflammatory mediators, including enzymes that can cause tissue damage. These cells have been shown to be potent effectors in killing invading parasites by antibody or complement dependent mechanisms. Eosinophils also play prominent roles in late-phase reactions that affect some people with allergies and asthma, particularly with symptoms of nasal congestion that can occur hours after an initial episode of allergic rhinitis. (See "Reacting to allergen exposures," later in this chapter.) If you have uncontrolled asthma, constant eosinophil activity may lead to *airway remodeling* — the replacement of healthy tissue with scar tissue — and can potentially cause irreversible loss of lung function.

Preventing this type of serious lung damage is one of the main goals of treating asthma early and aggressively, particularly with inhaled topical corticosteroids. Because eosinophils tend to accumulate in your nasal passages if you have allergic rhinitis, your doctor may use a nasal smear or a blood test (Chapter 8) to check for the presence of eosinophils when diagnosing your condition.

REMEMBER

Histamine and leukotrienes (which we refer to in many other parts of this book) are just two of the vast array of potent chemical mediators of inflammation released from mast cells and basophils during allergic reactions. This multitude of mediators can induce the following actions in your body:

>> Dilate your blood vessels, leading to increased fluid leakage, which increases inflammatory action.

>> Increase mucus secretions, resulting in a runny nose, watery eyes, and airway congestion, depending on where the trigger causes the allergic reaction.

>> Activate your sensory nerves, causing increased itching. (If you have allergic rhinitis, your nose may feel itchy when you experience other allergy symptoms because these mediators activate your sensory nerves.)

>> Cause tissue damage, often with accompanying pain and discomfort.

>> Promote the production of IgE and activation of eosinophils, thus supporting allergic inflammation.

>> Attract other inflammatory cells to the area to amplify the inflammatory reaction.

>> Cause constriction of the smooth muscles of your respiratory airways.

Reacting to allergen exposures

This section shows you how the players we describe in the preceding section interact. A typical sequence of reactions in an IgE response (immediate hypersensitivity) consists of the following steps:

1. **Your immune system receives exposure to an allergen.**

   Allergen exposures can result from the following occurrences:

   - **Inhaling:** Inhalant allergens (or *aeroallergens*) such as pollens, molds, dust mite allergens, and animal danders often pass through your nose and/or your mouth, throat, and airways of the lungs. Common symptoms of these exposures include runny nose, sneezing, watery eyes, stuffy nose, postnasal drip, coughing, chest tightness, wheezing, and shortness of breath.

   - **Ingesting:** You may swallow allergens, such those contained in peanuts, tree nuts, shellfish, eggs, milk, or in drugs such as penicillin. These exposures can trigger oral symptoms such as itching and swelling of the tongue, lips, and throat; GI tract symptoms such as nausea, stomach cramps, vomiting, and diarrhea; skin reactions such as hives and *angioedema* (deep swellings); and respiratory symptoms such as coughing, wheezing, stridor, and shortness of breath.

   - **Touching (direct contact):** Direct contact exposures typically involve Type IV delayed hypersensitivity responses, including reactions to poison ivy, nickel, and latex, among numerous others (Chapter 12). Symptoms from direct contact usually result in localized, topical reactions such as skin rashes.

   - **Injecting:** Medical syringes and insect stings and bites are vehicles for injecting allergens. Injections can cause particularly severe reactions because allergens go directly into your bloodstream, which can spread the allergens rapidly to organs throughout your body. Penicillin shots are the most dramatic (and often severe) examples of drug-related anaphylaxis in people with penicillin hypersensitivities. The venom from stinging insects can also cause potentially life-threatening reactions.

2. **Your body develops an IgE antibody response to the allergen.**

   If you have an atopic predisposition for developing allergies, scavenger cells (macrophages) that usually rid your body of foreign proteins (such as allergens) act as antigen- (allergen-) presenting cells (APCs). These APCs trigger T cells (other specialized immune system cells) to recruit B cells that develop into plasma cells. This process culminates in the production of specific IgE antibodies designed against the allergen (see Figure 2-1).

3. **Allergens bind to specific IgE antibodies attached to the surface of mast cells or basophils.**

   The first time you're exposed to the allergen, you don't typically experience a reaction. However, you produce specific IgE antibodies that bind to receptor sites on mast cells. Thus, your immune system is *sensitized,* and further exposure to that allergen initiates an allergic response.

4. **This cross-linking of the allergen to two specific IgE antibodies on the surface of the mast cell activates the mast cell to release its potent chemical mediators of inflammation, which affect various organs and trigger your allergic symptoms.**

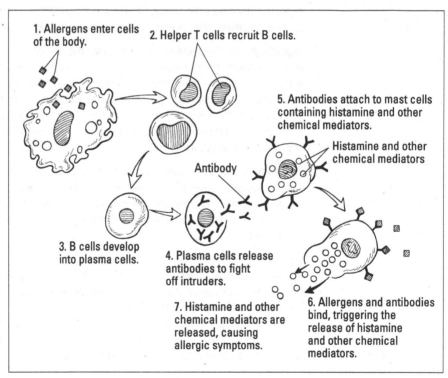

1. Allergens enter cells of the body.

2. Helper T cells recruit B cells.

3. B cells develop into plasma cells.

4. Plasma cells release antibodies to fight off intruders.

Antibody

5. Antibodies attach to mast cells containing histamine and other chemical mediators.

Histamine and other chemical mediators

6. Allergens and antibodies bind, triggering the release of histamine and other chemical mediators.

7. Histamine and other chemical mediators are released, causing allergic symptoms.

FIGURE 2-1:
The allergic inflammatory response is a complex process involving many types of cells.

In some cases, particularly with reactions to insects stings and penicillin, you many think that your allergic reaction was the result of just a single exposure. In most instances, however, you received a prior, sensitizing exposure, perhaps in one of the following ways:

- With regard to insect stings, you may have been stung as a child. If that experience wasn't traumatic and resulted only in a minor, localized reaction, you may have forgotten about it.

- Your first exposure to penicillin allergens may be even less memorable: the cow's milk or beef that you eat can include this antibiotic from the animal's feed.

Doing it one more time: The late-phase reaction

The allergic response consists of two phases involving inflammatory cells and potent chemical mediators of inflammation:

>> The immediate, early phase occurs within one hour of initial allergen exposure.

>> An additional, late-phase reaction, referred to as a *biphasic allergic reaction,* can occur in some people anywhere from three to ten hours after the initial allergic response.

Basophils influence eosinophils (see "Setting the stage for allergic reactions," earlier in this chapter) to stage a second, rallying effort against the allergen hours after you think you're recovered from an allergic episode. In some cases, this late-phase reaction can actually be more severe than the initial reaction. Congestion is often a prominent symptom of a late-phase response.

Because antihistamines and quick-relief bronchodilators are only effective for dealing with early-phase reactions, your doctor may need to prescribe oral corticosteroids (such as Prednisone or Medrol) to control late-phase symptoms. Immunotherapy is a unique form of treatment that helps decrease both early- and late-phased reactions to allergen exposures, as I explain in "Reaping the Benefits of Immunology," later in this chapter.

Becoming hyperresponsive

Typically, if you're consistently exposed to an indoor allergen — for instance, animal dander — you many find that during ragweed season, your symptoms appear to become more bothersome even at lower levels of exposure than you have experienced previously. By increasing your *allergen load* (your total level of exposure, at any one time, to any combination of allergens that trigger your allergies — see Chapter 5), other allergens and irritants may be more likely to also cause problems for you. In this case, eliminating animal dander from your home could result in fewer allergy symptoms during ragweed season.

Conversely, although your friend's cat might not be an issue for you most of the year, Fluffy's dander may trigger your allergic rhinitis and/or asthma symptoms during ragweed season. That's because exposure to the pollen causes you to develop a lower threshold for allergy symptoms (making you *hyperresponsive*) when exposed to this friendly feline.

Reacting non-specifically

Another reaction complication that occurs is non-specific-reactivity. *Non-specific reactivity* develops when your nasal passages and breathing airways become so inflamed and sensitized by repeated, constant exposure to triggering allergens that nonallergic irritants can also cause reactions. Non-specific irritants often include the following:

>> Tobacco smoke (from cigarettes, cigars, pipes, vapes)

>> Fumes and scents from household cleaners, strongly scented soaps, and perfumes and colognes; from glues, solvents, and aerosols; and from unvented gas, oil, or kerosene stoves

>> Smoke from wood-burning appliances or fireplaces

>> Air pollution

>> Gases, from chemicals found primarily in the workplace

WARNING

Although the reactions triggered by irritants aren't IGE-mediated, they still increase injury to already sensitive areas. If you're continuously exposed to allergens and irritants, a vicious cycle can develop, and the damage that allergic reactions cause is compounded by irritants, thus aggravating your affected areas further and increasing their sensitivities, resulting in more symptoms and further injury to your airways.

Reaping the Benefits of Immunology

Immunology provides great benefits for treating allergy and asthma conditions, enabling doctors to modify your immune system's reactions to allergy and asthma triggers with immunotherapy (also known as allergy shots). The immunologic response that results from immunotherapy triggers promotes immune system actions that protect rather than damage your body, as we discuss in Chapter 6.

Immunotherapy is the most effective way, in most cases, to treat the underlying causes of allergic ailments such as allergic rhinitis (and allergic conjunctivitis), allergic asthma, food allergies, and allergies to insect stings (with venom immunotherapy, or VIT, as we explain in Chapter 17).

DOCTOR SAYS

ENHANCING YOUR FUTURE WITH IMMUNOLOGY

The advances that medical science has made with immunology during the last century are among the greatest human achievements in the history of our species, producing medical miracles for the entire world that would have seemed like sheer fantasy 100 years ago. I believe that the continued progress in our understanding of immunology will enable medical researchers to find far more effective ways of preventing infectious diseases that continue to cause serious problems for many people around the world. Immunologic reseach has already helped control some forms of cancer with the use of interferons, anti-tumor antibody therapy, and other immunologic interventions.

In the quest for more effective medications to control allergy and asthma symptoms, immunology has been the key to developing a new and innovative medication, for example, based on using a high-tech antibody known as *recombinant human monoclonal antibody* (rhuMab), which is an anti-IgE antibody. This drug is designed to immunologically bind with circulating IgE. This binding prevents the binding of IgE to mast cells, thus blocking the initiation of the allergic reaction.

The study of immunology matters a great deal to the whole human race. As physicians and scientists, we must continue to advance our knowledge about our immune system and unlock the secrets it holds for a healthier future. The 21st century has seen the development of vaccines for many serious diseases such as herpes; respiratory syncytial virus (RSV) infections, which cause bronchiolitis in infants and potentially fatal pneumonia in adults (see Chapter 6); and the worldwide outbreak of COVID. Likewise, I think that the 21st century will also result in the development of more effective forms of immunotherapy for allergies. Immunologic research may one day even produce a vaccine against allergy and asthma.

Chapter **3**

Dealing With Physician Visits

Seeing a physician, whether an asthma or allergy specialist or your own family practitioner, is something you should prepare for each and every time you have an appointment. The two of you are partners in treating your medical condition. Developing and maintaining that partnership is one of the most important aspects of effectively managing and treating your allergies, asthma, or any other serious ailment. We often refer to this as *shared decision making,* and it's becoming more important in providing the best medical care.

TIP

The effectiveness of your treatment depends not so much on the *length* of time you spend in your physician's office, but rather on the *quality* of that time. As much as I (Dr. Berger) enjoy seeing my patients and as much as they may delight in my winning personality, the real reason they're in my office is to get better. In my experience, patients who derive the greatest benefit from treatment are those who understand how to get the most out of their physician visits. Some tips for getting the most include the following:

» Prepare ahead of time (as I explain in the next section of this chapter).

» Communicate well with your physician about your condition and the effects of your treatment.

» Understand all aspects of your treatment plan, including the medications that your physician prescribes, and learn the most effective ways of avoiding allergy and asthma triggers (Chapters 5 and 9 offer more information on avoiding allergy and asthma triggers).

» Participate in developing treatment goals with your physician and make sure that you can openly communicate with them about the effects and results of your treatment.

» Adhere to your treatment plan. You're the most important factor in your own treatment process. Your good health and your quality of life clearly depend on your full and active participation in the treatment process.

In this chapter we discuss what to expect during your first visit, including the questions your physician is likely to ask, and the types of tests they may perform to assist with an accurate diagnosis of your medical condition.

Preparing for Your First Visit

When it comes to making a proper diagnosis of allergies and asthma, your primary care physician may refer you to a specialist, such as an allergist (see the nearby sidebar) and/or a pulmonologist (lung doctor). Your first visit will most likely cover the following items:

» Taking a thorough medical history (see the next sections), covering any and all ailments in your life, not just those that you think involve allergies or asthma.

» Performing a physical examination. Depending on your condition, your past medical history, and especially on why your primary care physician referred you, your physical exam may focus only on the areas that your allergy or asthma symptoms affect, or if indicated, your exam may also include a more comprehensive evaluation. (Refer to the section "Looking for signs of asthma and allergies" later in this chapter for more information on the signs and symptoms your doctor may be looking for, depending on your medical history.)

» Allergy skin testing (depending on your medical history and medical exam) for specific allergic sensitivities and/or other appropriate tests and lab procedures (such as pulmonary function tests for asthma, as we explain in "Assessing asthma with spirometry" later in this chapter).

» Prescribing and teaching you how to use appropriate medications and/or instructing you about effective environmental control steps that you can take to avoid or reduce exposure to your allergy or asthma triggers, thus reducing symptoms.

SEEING A SPECIALIST

We recommend that you or your physician consider consulting an asthma and allergy specialist, such as an allergist or pulmonologist (lung doctor), when:

- **Your diagnosis is difficult to establish.** Chronic coughing and/or a runny nose that don't respond to initial treatment, such as cough or cold medications, are two of the most frequent reasons why your primary care physician may refer you to an asthma and allergy specialist.

- **Your diagnosis requires specialized testing.** In some cases, your primary care physician may refer you to specialist for allergy skin testing to confirm their suspicion of an underlying allergy, such as *allergic rhinitis* (hay fever), asthma, *atopic dermatitis* (eczema), hypersensitivities to certain foods, or allergic insect sting reactions. Other types of specialized tests that involve referring you to a specialist and include diagnostic procedures for asthma, such as spirometry or complete pulmonary function studies, bronchoprovocation or bronchoscopy (see Chapter 8), and/or further evaluation of your rhinitis with rhinoscopy. In addition, your physician may recommend an oral food challenge to help diagnose possible food allergy.

- **Your physician advises you to consider *immunotherapy* (allergy shots).** See Chapter 4 for more information on immunotherapy.

- **Other conditions complicate your condition or its diagnosis.** Those conditions may include sinusitis, nasal polyps, severe rhinitis gastroesophageal reflux disease (GERD), chronic obstructive pulmonary disease (COPD), vocal cord dysfunction (VCD), or aspergillosis (a fungal infection that can affect your lungs).

- **You've experienced a previous emergency room visit or hospitalization for asthma (see Chapter 8), food allergy, or anaphylaxis (see Chapter 15).**

Doing your homework

Identifying the underlying cause of your allergy or asthma provides the best approach to effectively treating your ailment. However, as we explain in Chapter 2, because of the complexity of allergic diseases, getting to the root of what's ailing you is usually more than a matter of just performing medical tests (such as blood tests or X-rays) and interpreting the results.

Although we've seen impressive breakthroughs recently in diagnosing and treating various diseases (especially with ongoing research in developing new medications), the first step an allergy or asthma specialist still takes to treat your condition is obtaining your complete medical history. The specialist uses your medical history as the foundation of your medical evaluation.

The physician you're consulting for your allergy and/or asthma condition usually requests that you provide very specific medical information at your first visit. After taking your medical history, your specialist may also perform and appropriate medical exam. Subsequently they may also order tests and procedures to confirm your diagnosis and to identify the specific triggers of your allergy symptoms more precisely, as well as to determine your sensitivity levels to those triggers.

TIP

Preparing for an initial consultation with a specialist shouldn't stress you out the way school exams or job interviews may sometimes affect you. However you need to spend some time before your appointment gathering and reviewing information that your specialist needs in order to make a specific diagnosis of your condition. Prepare to provide them with and to discuss in detail during your consultation the following key information:

>> Your symptoms, both those that seems to be caused by an allergic condition and any others you may be experiencing, even if they seem unrelated.

>> Any other medical conditions for which you've been treated or are presently being treated.

>> Any medications you're taking, whether prescription or over-the counter (OTC).

>> Your medical history, as well as that of your family.

>> Details about other factors, such as your home, work, or school environment, that may contribute to your medical condition.

We provide detailed examples that your physician will request, based on these general categories, in the next section of this chapter. You may also have questions about your medical condition. Asking your physician about your concerns during your initial consultation is certainly appropriate. Remember, there's no such thing as a stupid question when you're asking about your medical history, diagnosis, or treatment.

REMEMBER

You may think that an issue you raise is obvious, insignificant, or irrelevant, but bringing it up may further clarify the nature of your ailment. The best way to ding out is to go ahead and ask. A good physician appreciates the fact that you've taken the time to formulate your own questions. We advise writing down your inquiries ahead of time and giving them to your physician at the beginning of your appointment, so that they can focus on the most important issues affecting your health during your office visit.

Filling out forms ahead of time

Many physicians (including me, Dr. Berger) send patients a questionnaire to fill out prior to their initial consultation. The level of detail that these questionnaires require varies, depending on the symptoms you experience and the type of consultation you seek. Physicians don't send out these forms because they love paperwork, but rather because they want to ensure that your first appointment is most productive.

TIP

In most cases, you can expect to spend between one and two hours at your first appointment. You may have a hectic life, but plan your schedule so that you can arrive at your physician's office on time or even a few minutes early. Remember to bring all requested forms, documents, and other materials, including your insurance and/or other payment information. (Refer to the section "Paying for Your Care" later in this chapter.)

Telling your story

Whatever way it's gathered, you need to provide the following information at your first appointment with your asthma and allergy specialist:

- » Your name, address, email, telephone number, and other contact information.

- » You age, gender, and occupation. (If you're making an appointment for your child, list your own and your partner's age and occupation.)

- » The name of your referring physician (or other person who referred you).

- » The symptoms you're experiencing and the specific areas or organs of your body that are affected. (Providing details of when and in what circumstances these symptoms occur is often vital to establishing an accurate diagnosis).

- » For women, let your physician know if you think or know you're pregnant or if you're planning to become pregnant.

- » Aggravating factors that seem to make your condition worse. For example, if you notice that your respiratory symptoms — such as coughing, wheezing, or shortness of breath — are more severe when you visit people who have pets or when you're around smokers, make sure you tell your physician.

- » The names of all the medications you're currently taking, including products that you use specifically for your conditions, as well as other drugs, such as OTC preparations or herbal remedies, which you take to relieve minor aches and pains. (We advise bringing a list of medications you're currently taking.) If you're unsure of the actual drugs that you use (perhaps the label is difficult to decipher), bring the medication with you in it is original container. Also, ask your pharmacist, primary care physician, or other doctors for a list of medications they've prescribed for any of your medical conditions. Because gathering this information all at once can be a challenge, we advise keeping a drug record that you can refer to when consulting with a new doctor, as we explain in the section "Recording your symptoms and medication" later in this chapter.

>> If you've been treated or evaluated previously for the same condition, provide your new physician with information on the results of these consultations and treatments. (Bringing the results from any tests you have in the past may also save you the trouble — and cost — of repeating those procedures.)

Providing accurate information on any other illnesses and related treatments you've have is also vital to evaluating your current condition.

>> Your family history is very important in determining your diagnosis, so take time to list this information to the best of your ability (see the section "Taking your family history" later in this chapter). Likewise, if you fill out this form for a child, provide information on specific childhood factors, such as birth history (including gestational age), immunizations, and childhood illnesses (for example, bronchiolitis and/or or croup).

>> Your career, occupation, the school (or daycare for children) you attend, and your hobbies or recreational activities are also important factors in figuring out what's ailing you.

>> Your dietary history, including any special diets you follow, major food groups you avoid, and whether you've been diagnosed with any food allergies or sensitivities.

Physicians aren't census-takers (or private detectives, for that matter), but your specialist needs to know about your home because many things there can trigger or aggravate allergy and/or asthma symptoms, particularly dust, animal dander, molds, and tobacco smoke. Therefore, you should provide your physician with information on the following items:

>> A list of people living with you and any habits they may have, such as smoking or keeping pets, that can affect your condition.

>> If you have plants in your home, identify them for your physician.

>> In addition, although specialists also aren't contractors, real estate agents, architects, or interior decorators, they generally try to assess the condition of your home including its location, age, the principal construction materials, the building's air circulation system, the condition of the basement, and the type of carpets and furnishings you have. Your physician may also ask about your yard, garden, and surrounding vegetation.

>> Your physician usually asks about your bedroom also. Don't worry; they aren't getting personal. However, because the bedroom is where you most likely spend the majority of your life (even more time than on the golf course, in

Dr. Berger's case), exposure to allergens in your bedroom can often play a significant role in the severity of your allergy or asthma symptoms.

>> Some patients want to record the conversation at their physician visit using the voice recorder on their smartphone. They feel that doing so allows them to listen to the visit over again in case they missed something or didn't understand the first time, what was being recommended. However, privacy and confidentiality are the cornerstones of the physician-patient relationship; therefore, everyone in the exam room including the physician and other medical team members must be made aware of the recording and provide permission to having the discussion recorded.

Recording your symptoms and medications

Keeping a daily symptom diary can provide valuable information that your physician can use when assessing your condition. A typical daily symptom diary is usually a table with columns and rows where you can record items, such as your daily symptoms, medications you take, your peak expiratory flow rate (PEFR, to monitor asthma; see Chapter 10), and your observations about possible triggers or suspected exposures.

REMEMBER

In addition to keeping a symptom diary, we also recommend establishing a medication record that lists all the drugs — prescription, OTC, and herbal remedies — that you take over your lifetime. Recording your medications is similar to recording checks in your check register.

TIP

PATIENT, KNOW THYSELF

Providing your physician with the information that they request about your medical history enables you to take part in the process of diagnosing and treating your medical problems, often referred to as *shared decision making*. While assembling their medical histories and related details, many of my patients have discovered patterns and connections between symptoms, triggers, and precipitating factors that they hadn't realized before.

Gaining this type of self-knowledge not only helps your physicians make a diagnosis, but it also helps you make better choices about your treatment as well assist you in avoiding the triggers and precipitating factors of your allergies or asthma.

If you think that you may suffer from drug hypersensitivity (see Chapter 16), this medication record can also greatly help your physician diagnose the problem. Your medication record should include the brand and generic names of *all* drugs you've used and currently take, including OTC vitamins and supplements — some of which are as potent as conventional medical products that the Food and Drug Administration (FDA) regulates and that are available only by prescription. In addition, you should also note the conditions you treat or have treated with particular drugs and the effectiveness and/or results of taking those products.

Focusing on foods

In addition to causing digestive problems such as nausea, vomiting, or diarrhea, *hypersensitivities* (allergies) to certain foods can trigger symptoms throughout your body. Food hypersensitivity symptoms can include stuffy nose, skin rashes and hives, headaches, respiratory problems (such as coughing, wheezing, and shortness of breath), and general fatigue. Symptoms may occur rapidly after eating the food or may be delayed.

If your physician suspects that food hypersensitivity causes your symptoms, they may advise you to keep a detailed food diary to bring to your initial specialist consultation. Your food diary can help your specialist determine whether or not your problem is a food allergy or the result of another type of adverse food reaction, such as a food intolerance (see Chapter 15 for information on keeping a food diary). You should also tell your doctor about any foods you may be avoiding due to a suspected food allergy or intolerance.

Taking your family history

Because heredity often plays an important role in determining your likelihood of developing allergies, your physician usually asks about your family medical history. You don't need to become a private investigator or a Sherlock Holmes to research this information, but you should make sure that you know which relative (mother, brother, uncle, and so on) had a particular disease or condition. Letting your physician know whether your parents, siblings or close relatives had allergic conditions such as asthma, allergic rhinitis, atopic dermatitis, and food or drug allergies is important.

Looking for signs of asthma and allergies

After discussing your medical history, your physician will probably examine you for physical signs of your allergies or asthma. The areas that they usually check vary based on your medical history, as well as the type of symptoms you have. Areas that they many investigate include the following:

>> Eyes, ears, nose, throat, and sinuses. Physicians often check for redness and watering of eyes; appearance of your eardrums; swelling of your nasal lining; amount and character of nasal discharge; presence of nasal polyps; size and color of tonsils; tender or swollen lymph nodes in your neck area; and possible tenderness over your sinus areas.

>> Your chest and torso, to look for expanded or over-inflated lugs and hunched shoulders, which can signal breathing difficulties.

>> Your lungs (with a stethoscope). To check for wheezing, other abnormal breath sounds, and the character of your airflow.

>> Your skin, to check for dry, red, itchy, and damaged skin (as is seen in atopic dermatitis), which may indicate your predisposition to allergies.

>> If your physician suspects allergic rhinitis as part of your problem, they may also look for distinctive combinations of gestures and facial features, particularly in children and adolescents, as we detail in Chapter 4.

Allergy testing and other diagnostic studies

In order to confirm or more precisely identify and underlying cause of your symptoms, your physician may advise certain tests and procedures. The types of diagnostic studies that your specialist performs depend on your medical history and the results of your physical examination. In the following sections, we provide an overview of the most frequently used tests and procedures.

Allergy skin testing

Allergists consider skin testing the gold standard for identifying sensitivities to certain types of allergens. In some cases, allergy skin testing can also indicate your level of sensitivity to the particular allergen. Allergy skin tests are usually most useful for identifying sensitivities to pollen, dust mites, molds, animal dander, insect stings, food hypersensitivities, and if necessary, for penicillin hypersensitivities.

TECHNICAL
STUFF

Skin testing for allergies in the specialist's office generally involves placing a drop of a suspected allergen on your skin and then pricking, puncturing, or scratching your skin with a device to see whether the allergen produces a reaction. If you're allergic to the administered allergen, your skin usually reacts in a way that resembles a mosquito bite or small hive.

A positive reaction can help identify the cause of your allergic reactions and may also indicate your sensitivity level to that allergic trigger. (Refer to Chapter 4 to find out more about allergy skin testing.)

Using *ImmunoCAP* for allergy testing

Your allergist may recommend using ImmunoCAP for diagnosing your allergic sensitivities. This blood test uses fluorescently labeled detection antibodies to measure levels of specific IgEs. Although ImmunoCAP isn't as precise, practical, comprehensive, or cost-effective as allergy skin testing, your physician may advise using this procedure under specific circumstances. See Chapter 4 for more information on ImmunoCAP.

Assessing asthma with spirometry

If your symptoms include coughing, wheezing, and shortness of breath, your physician should assess your lung functions with spirometry to evaluate whether asthma is the underlying cause of your condition.

TECHNICAL STUFF

A *spirometer* is a sophisticated machine that measure airflow from your large and small airways before and after you inhale a short-acting bronchodilator. For adults and children over age 4 or 5, this procedure provides the most accurate way of determining whether airway obstruction exists and whether your condition is reversible (meaning that it improves after taking appropriate medication). Your physician may also advise other lung function tests if they suspect that other coexisting respiratory conditions may cause or affect your symptoms (see Chapter 8).

Other procedures for diagnosing allergies and asthma

Confirming an allergy or asthma diagnosis may also involve additional studies and tests, such as:

>> **Rhinoscopy:** This technique is useful for investigating causes of nasal obstruction or blockage, postnasal drainage, and the condition of the sinuses.

>> **Nasal smear:** Although not considered a definitive diagnostic test, a nasal smear can help your physician determine whether you suffer from allergic rhinitis. This procedure generally involves taking secretions from your nose, usually with a flexible, plastic device, which your physician then examines under a microscope for levels of *eosinophils* (at type of white blood cell — see Chapter 2). Elevated counts of eosinophils can indicate an allergic condition.

>> **Blood tests:** Your physician may also order an IgE level to screen for allergy and a blood eosinophil count to help characterize the nature of your asthma and to determine what treatment might be best for your medical condition.

>> **A chest and/or sinus X-ray or a CT scan of the sinuses (see Chapter 7):** Your physician may also order these types of imaging tests to determine whether other disorders, such as chronic bronchitis and emphysema — collectively referred to as *chronic obstructive pulmonary disease (COPD)*, pneumonia, or sinusitis (sinus infection) may be part of your medical condition.

>> **Bronchoprovocation:** In some cases, spirometry may indicate normal or near-normal lung functions, although asthma nonetheless seems the most likely cause of your symptoms. Therefore, your physician may advise broncho-provocation to diagnose your condition more precisely. These types of tests usually involve exercising for several minutes (on a stationary bicycle or treadmill in your physician's office) or inhaling a small dose of methacholine or histamine, in order to determine whether mild asthma symptoms occur as a result of bronchial constriction. This test allows physicians to diagnose individuals whose asthma is otherwise not apparent, but whose symptoms appear as a response to these challenges due to the hyperreactivity of their airways (see Chapter 8).

>> **Tympanometry:** Physicians often use this procedure, which measures your ear drum response to various pressure levels, to determine whether you have *otitis media* (inflammation of the middle ear, often associated with ear infections) — a frequent complication of both sinusitis and allergic rhinitis.

>> **Thyroid function test:** Because *hypothyroidism* (an underactive thyroid) can cause chronic nasal congestion similar to a severe case of allergic rhinitis, your physician may order this test to rule out an alternative diagnosis.

WARNING

>> **Elimination diet:** If skin testing for food allergies isn't conclusive, your physician may advise an elimination diet (which you should only undertake under your physician's supervision) to confirm what's triggering your adverse food reactions. (For more food for thought on food allergies, turn to Chapter 15.)

WARNING

>> **Oral food challenges:** These tests involve ingesting — under medical supervision — increasing amounts of very small quantities of foods that contain suspected allergens. They should be performed only if your previous adverse food reactions haven't been life-threatening (see Chapter 15).

Following Up: Second and Subsequent Visits

Your second visit with an allergy or asthma specialist usually takes place one to two weeks after your initial consultation. This return visit is every bit as important as your first appointment, so make sure that you take with you any information, records, or documents your physician may require, based on your previous appointment. Here we discuss what you can expect.

TIP

When scheduling your follow-up visit, we suggest asking your physician's office how much time the physician expects to spend with you, so you can plan your day accordingly.

Doctor, doctor, give me the news

During your second consultation, your physician usually goes over the results of your tests, explains your diagnosis, and reviews your treatment plan. This follow-up visit is often referred to as a *summary conference*.

TIP

Depending on your diagnosis and medical condition, your physician may take all or some of the following steps during your second visit (or third visit in some cases):

>> **Review the effectiveness of medications that they prescribed for you at your previous visit.** In some cases your physician may need to adjust your medications and dosages.

>> **Provide you with a summary of the most important findings of your initial consultation.** You should also ask for recommendations concerning additional educational materials (such as this book!).

>> **Provide with a written treatment plan.** Make sure that you understand this plan and can adhere to it. If you have concerns or questions about your advised treatment, inform your physician.

>> **Give you handouts with written instructions on avoiding the allergens, irritants, and/or precipitating factors that may trigger your asthma or allergies.** Make sure to read these instructions carefully after your visit and follow up with your physician if you have any questions or if anything is unclear.

Considering allergy shots

If your medical history and skin testing provide clear evidence that you're allergic to certain allergens, your physician may advise you to consider immunotherapy. If they suggest immunotherapy, they should make sure that you understand the commitment this treatment requires.

REMEMBER

Immunotherapy isn't a quick fix, and it requires a significant investment of time on your part. For inhalant allergens and insect stings (using venom immuno-therapy, or VIT, as we explain in Chapter 17), it may take up to one year of allergy shots before you and your doctor can determine whether you're clearly benefitting from the therapy. Your adherence to the program is the key for effective immuno-therapy, meaning that you need to maintain the injection schedule that your allergist prescribes as much a possible (see Chapter 4).

Paying for Your Care

Here's the fun part: dealing with medical bills. Make sure you read and under-stand your physician's office financial policy before your first appointment so that you know and understand what your payment terms are.

REMEMBER

The terms of financial policies usually depend on the level and type of health insurance you carry. If you're covered by Medicare or a contracted insurance plan, such as a health maintenance organization (HMO), you generally aren't billed, although you many need to make a small co-payment at the time of your visit (usually between $5 and $20).

However, you many need to pay out-of-pocket for your first office visit (at the time of your appointment) if any of the following applies to you:

>> You don't carry health insurance.

>> You don't have a private health insurance policy.

>> You aren't covered by an insurance plan, such as an HMO, that contracts with your doctor's practice.

>> You can't (or don't) provide your doctor's office with insurance information. (Make sure you have all requested healthcare documents and records with you when you see your physician.)

Dealing with insurance issues

With the movement toward managed care, seeing a specialist is frequently more difficult for patients. Consider discussing your needs with the human resources specialist in your workplace or an independent insurance broker who can help you find a plan that provides access to the physicians you need to see, when you need to see them, is preferable. If you have the opportunity to choose among several medical coverage plans, paying a little bit more for a policy that allows direct access to specialists when you need them is well worth the extra investment. (Just like with most other purchases, you get what you pay for!)

DOCTOR SAYS

I strongly advise my patients not to sell themselves short by buying insurance solely on the basis of price. A low-cost plan may work just fine when you're in good health and don't really require much specialty medical care. However, if you develop a serious medical problem, you may find that many of these low-cost plans cover expert treatment only after your ailment deteriorates into a potentially irreversible or life-threatening condition.

Gatekeeping and your treatment

Good primary care practitioners on the front lines of health are essential to the well-being of much of the world's population, especially in the United States. In the United States, however, these physicians often work under difficult circumstances because of the limitations and deficiencies of the health insurance financing system.

In many cases, HMOs attempt to control their costs by providing bonuses and other incentives to primary care physicians (often known as *gatekeepers*) who limit referrals to specialists. *Capitation*, which involves giving these physicians restricted budgets for treating patients, has led to many complaints by both patients and primary care physicians alike.

According to a study in the *New England Journal of Medicine*, at least one-quarter of primary care physicians worry that they're treating complicated conditions that specialists could handle better. This study also found that many primary care physicians, who receive a larger proportion of their income through capitation and who serve as gatekeepers for large numbers of patients, think their practice is too broad. These physicians also report that they're often required to treat people with more complex conditions than they treated in the past.

Getting the care you need and deserve

If your primary care physician tells you that no other treatment is available for your condition, they may really mean that nothing more can be done for you in your managed care setting. If this situation happens to you and/or you're dissatisfied with the medical care you're receiving, consider doing the following:

>> **Find out whether your HMO provides bonuses or other forms of incentives for limiting referrals.** Although you many feel uncomfortable asking your primary care physician about this topic, you have a right to know about the policies that directly affect the delivery of your healthcare.

>> **Become your own advocate.** Read up on the current issues regarding healthcare and understand your rights (as well as your responsibilities) as a patient. Especially if your child has asthma, an excellent place to start is by reading *A Parent's Guide to Asthma: How You Can Help Your Child Control Asthma at Home, School, and Play* by my friend Nancy Sander, the founder of the Allergy and Asthma Network/Mothers of Asthmatics.

>> **If a managed care plan that you're considering lists an impressive roster of specialists, make sure you can consult with these experts when you need them.** Some HMOs won't let you see a specialist until you're hospitalized, which is one hospitalization too many.

Working Well with Your Physician

Expectations from treatment can vary from one individual to another, often depending on different people's priorities in life, so make sure you clearly communicate your own personal expectations to your physician. Ask what you should expect to achieve from the treatment they prescribe for you and participate in setting and developing your own individualized treatment goals. (If you have asthma, see the suggested goals for an effective asthma management plan, which we list in Chapter 8.)

TIP

The vast majority of people with asthma and allergies can lead normal lives. With effective, appropriate care from your physician and your own motivated participation as a patient, your treatment plan should enable you to lead a full and active life. However, if following your plan properly doesn't allow you to participate fully in the activities and pursuits that matter to you, openly communicate your concerns to your physician and together adjust your plan to maximize the effectiveness of your treatment.

2

Knowing Your Nose

IN THIS PART . . .

Understand the need for a medical evaluation to determine what's ailing your nose.

Investigate inhalant allergens that might be adversely affecting your sinuses.

Avoid environmental allergies that trigger your nasal symptoms.

Allergy-proof your home and bedroom.

Know your pharmacology choices to manage sinusitis effectively.

Understand common nasal allergy complications such as worsening asthma, bronchitis, otitis media, and nasal polyps.

Chapter **4**

Nosing Around Allergic Rhinitis

llergic rhinitis, more commonly referred to as *hay fever,* is the most common allergic disease in the United States. As many as 50 to 80 million Americans may suffer from some form of this allergy, including 10 to 30 percent of all adults and up to 40 percent of all children. That's a lot of sneezing fits, runny noses, clogged sinuses, and itchy, watery eyes. Although the effects of allergic rhinitis are rarely life-threatening (even though you sometimes feel as if you could die when the symptoms take hold), allergic rhinitis can still be a debilitating disease with serious consequences if you don't treat and manage it appropriately.

REMEMBER

The term *hay fever* is actually a misnomer, stemming from the 19th century studies of English farmers who mistakenly blamed spring hay cutting as the cause of nasal inflammatory ailments. Likewise, people in the 19th century referred to any ailment as a fever. In 1871 Charles H. Blackley identified airborne pollen from various plants — especially grasses — that depend on wind for cross-pollination as the primary causes. The term "grass grief" didn't catch on, however, so the term *hay fever* is still used as a generic term for *allergic rhinitis* — usually for the most common variety, *seasonal allergic rhinitis.*

Allergic rhinitis affects so many people that the estimated costs of medical treatment, absenteeism, and lost productivity from this type of allergy are perhaps as high as $11 billion annually in the United States. Furthermore, allergic rhinitis results in 3.8 million lost workdays and 2 million lost school days annually. The cost per person with allergic rhinitis can exceed $1,000 annually, which further highlights the financial burden for both the individual and the healthcare system.

Studies have shown that 80 percent of people with allergic rhinitis develop the condition before their 20th birthday. U.S. schoolchildren with allergic rhinitis are at an increased risk of experiencing developmental delays (such as hearing and speech difficulties); suffering from poor school performance (due to drowsiness and irritability); and developing learning disabilities (due to poor focus and concentration), as well as emotional and behavioral problems.

RHINOIDS, RHINITIS, AND RHINOS: IT'S ALL GREEK TO YOUR NOSE

Rhinitis is the medical term for inflammation of the nasal mucous membranes. The word derives from the *rhin*, the ancient Greek for nose — hence the rhinoceros with horns (*keros*) on its nose — but has no relation to the Rhine, although your nose may run like a river during allergy season.

The second part of the terms, *itis*, means swelling or inflammation, as in *tonsillitis* (an inflammation of the tonsils), or *appendicitis* (an inflammation of the appendix), and of course — you guessed it — *rhinitis*, an inflamed nose.

Here's some more nosy terminology that you can use to impress your friends and to better understand your doctor:

- **Rhinology:** The anatomy, pathology, and physiology of the nose.
- **Rhinoscopy:** An examination of your nasal passages.
- **Rhinovirus:** A virus that causes respiratory disorders such as the common cold.
- **Rhinopharyngitis:** An inflammation that affects the mucous membranes of the nose and throat.
- **Rhinorrhea:** Runny nose.

SEE YOUR DOCTOR
Although often called hay fever, allergic rhinitis itself doesn't cause a fever. If you do run a temperature while experiencing symptoms that resemble hay fever, you may actually be suffering from a viral or bacterial infection, such sinusitis (see Chapter 7), influenza (flu), or pneumonia.

Catching Up with Your Runny Nose

REMEMBER

In order to effectively and appropriately manage allergic rhinitis, we strongly advise you to consider the following factors:

>> **You're in it for the long term:** This disease usually recurs persistently and indefinitely after you've become sensitized to the *allergens* (see Chapter 5) that trigger allergic rhinitis symptoms.

>> **You need a healthy nose:** Because your nose is such a vital part of your respiratory system, nasal health is vital to your overall wellness. Lack of treatment or ineffective or inappropriate management of allergic rhinitis can lead to complications such as nasal polyps (outgrowths of the nasal lining), sinusitis (inflammation of the sinuses), recurrent ear infections (potentially causing hearing loss; see Chapter 7 for both), aggravation of bronchial symptoms, dental and facial abnormalities, and poor speech development in children. Not only does your nose hold your sunglasses, but it also provides other beneficial functions:

- Your nose helps to warm and humidify the air you breathe in.

- The interior of your nose acts to filter and cleanse the air your breathe in, through the action of the *cilia* (tiny hair-like cells that sweep mucus through the nose).

- Your nose is also critical for your sense of small and the quality of your voice. For example, when your nose is stuffy or congested, your voice often sounds different (often referred to as *nasal voice*).

>> **You need to know why you're blowing your nose:** A proper diagnosis of your allergic rhinitis condition requires a review of your medical history, a physical examination, observation, analysis, and, in some cases, skin testing to identify the allergens involved, all to help determine the most effective course of treatment.

>> **Avoidance may be the key:** In many cases, the most effective and least expensive method of managing your allergic rhinitis is to avoid the allergens that trigger your symptoms. Although you may not be able to completely avoid all the allergens that cause your symptoms, partial avoidance may

provide you with enough relief to substantially improve your quality of life (see Chapter 5 for avoidance information).

>> **Drugs can be dangerous:** If you suffer from allergic rhinitis, you may resort to common first-generation, over-the-counter (OTC) antihistamines, decongestants, and nasal sprays to relieve your symptoms. However, many of these medications, often produce significant side effects, including drowsiness (seriously limiting the safe use of these antihistamines), impaired vision, hypertension, nausea, gastric distress, constipation, insomnia, irritability — and that's the short list. Besides creating more havoc in your life that allergic rhinitis already causes, these side effects can also be potentially dangerous. Overusing OTC decongestant nasal sprays can also lead to a condition known as *nasal rebound* (see Chapter 6).

Intranasal antihistamines (nasal sprays such as azelastine (Astepro) and olopatadine (Patanol) are recommended as first line treatments for seasonal and perennial allergic rhinitis and are thought to be more effective in managing associated nasal congestion and are faster acting than oral antihistamines.

>> **New and improved medications are available:** In cases where avoidance doesn't provide you with sufficient relief, newer and safer prescription drugs — including second-generation nonsedating and less-sedating antihistamines and nasal sprays — are often effective and produce fewer side effects than their OTC counterparts. However, these prescription drugs are only effective if you follow your physician's instructions and take them properly.

FEAR OF FLOWERS: ROSE FEVER AND OTHER NOSE MISNOMERS

Roses, like hay, receive a bad rap. Because these flowers tend to bloom in spring and summer when levels of windborne tree and grass pollens are usually at their peak, some allergic rhinitis sufferers mistakenly blame roses for causing allergy symptoms (hence the term *rose fever*). However, insects pollinate most attractive, colorful plants, including roses. In contrast to lighter tree, weed, and grass pollen and mold spores, the pollen that these plants produce is a sticky, heavier pollen that's much less likely to become windborne.

In fact, among the more than 700 species of North American trees, only about 10 percent release pollens that trigger symptoms of allergic rhinitis. Please note, however, that if you're a gardener and/or a florist who maintains a consistently high exposure to many types of flowers (not just roses), you can become sensitized to pollen from flowering plants, resulting in a form of occupational allergic rhinitis.

Naming the Types of Allergic Rhinitis

Hay fever is a common and nonspecific term for many varied types of allergic rhinitis, and it's often used in a general manner when discussing nasal inflammatory disorders — as well as for selling hay fever medications. Because the term *hay fever* describes so many different nasal inflammatory disorders, you may not be aware that allergists make distinctions between the different forms of allergic rhinitis. Allergists group these forms of hay fever according to the various types and patterns of exposure.

Here are the three principal classifications of allergic rhinitis, which the following sections discuss in greater detail:

>> Seasonal allergic rhinitis

>> Perennial allergic rhinitis, including perennial allergic rhinitis with seasonal exacerbation (worsening — see the nearby sidebar for more information)

>> Occupational allergic rhinitis

Seasonal allergic rhinitis

Seasonal allergic rhinitis is the most common form of allergic rhinitis, with symptoms occurring at specific times of the year when particular pollen and/or mold spore allergens are in the air. Symptoms can vary from year to year, however due to climactic conditions and regional differences that affect the quality and quantity of pollen and mold spores in the environment. Symptoms can also vary because of the timing and types of exposure that you experience to these substances. The levels of windborne tree, grass, and weed pollens are usually at their peak in the United States and Canada during the following times of year:

>> **Late winder (warmer climates) to late spring:** Tree pollens.

>> **Late spring to early summer:** Grass pollens.

>> **Mid-summer to fall:** Weed pollens, especially ragweed, which accounts for up to three-quarters of seasonal allergic rhinitis cases in the United States. The presence of weed pollen may continue in warmer climates through December, in the absence of an early frost.

REMEMBER

Windborne mold spores are present at various levels for most of the year, but they tend to cause a significant problem mostly during the late summer and fall. For more details on what's blowin' in the wind, turn to Chapter 5.

Perennial allergic rhinitis

Perennial allergic rhinitis is usually the result of your immune system becoming sensitized to a triggering agent or combination of agents that are constantly present in the environment, whether in the home, outdoors, at work or school, or other locations that you frequent. The symptoms involved in this condition can be just as severe as the symptoms of seasonal allergic rhinitis.

Occupational allergic rhinitis

Occupational allergic rhinitis is more difficult to diagnose and treat, because it often involves various combinations of a multitude of potential triggering agents and irritants found in many workplaces and occupations. Also, this specific type of allergic rhinitis often affects people with occupational asthma. (We provide details on occupational asthma in Chapter 8.) Your physician should determine the following factors in the course of diagnosing occupational allergic rhinitis:

>> Do your symptoms primarily occur at work? Or, if already present elsewhere, do your symptoms worsen while in the workplace?

>> Do your symptoms disappear or improve after you leave work — at the end of the day; during weekends or vacations, when your work location changes; or if you take a new job?

>> Do any of your colleagues and coworkers experience similar allergic symptoms?

Exploring What Makes Noses Run

In addition to windborne grass, weed, and tree pollens and mold spores, other allergic and nonallergic rhinitis triggers found in indoor environments include

>> Dust mite allergens

>> Indoor mold growths

>> Animal dander, saliva, and urine from warm-blooded pets such as dogs and cats

>> Waste and remains of pests, such as mice, rats, and cockroaches

>> Allergens found in workplaces, schools, or other indoor or enclosed locations that you frequent

>> Allergenic substances, such as fibers, latex, wood dust, various chemicals, and many other items

As we explain in Chapter 2, many substances that don't trigger an allergic response from your body's immune system can still intensify allergy or asthma conditions. Allergists refer to these substances as *irritants.* Common types of irritants include tobacco smoke, aerosols, glue, household cleaners, perfumes and scents, and strongly scented soaps.

Getting a Medical Evaluation

SEE YOUR DOCTOR

We strongly advise anyone who experiences significant hay fever symptoms to consult a physician to determine whether those symptoms are the result of a form of allergic rhinitis, a nonallergic type of rhinitis, a sinus infection, or a respiratory disease. A proper diagnosis is critical for the effective and appropriate management of any of the following conditions.

That sneezy, itchy, runny feeling

Many allergic rhinitis sufferers mistakenly assume that they have lingering colds that afflict them every spring (or whenever the weather changes). However, even though viral infections such as the common cold and various strains of flu may follow cyclical patterns, the frequency of these illnesses usually isn't as consistent or as constant as seasonal, perennial, or occupational allergic rhinitis. Symptoms associated with these forms of allergic rhinitis may often include

>> Runny nose with clear, watery discharge

>> Nasal congestion (stuffy nose)

>> Sneezing

>> Postnasal drip (nasal discharge down the back of your throat)

>> Itchy, watery eyes (allergic conjunctivitis)

>> Itchy, nose, ears, and throat

>> Persistent irritation of the mucous membranes of the eyes, middle ear, nose, and sinuses (in chronic cases).

Approximately half of all patients with allergic rhinitis experience additional clinical symptoms due to a *late-phase reaction*, occurring three to ten hours after allergen exposure, which typically leads to persistent symptoms, especially nasal congestion. The late-phase reaction is also implicated in *nonspecific reactivity* (increased sensitivity) of the nasal lining to nonallergic irritants (see Chapter 2).

SEE YOUR DOCTOR

Allergic rhinitis usually does *not* cause symptoms such as fever, achy muscles or joints, or tooth or eye pain. If you're experiencing these types of symptoms, the source of your ailment may be a type of viral or bacterial infection or the result of some physical factor, such as injury. Your physician should evaluate your condition.

TIP

If you have a deviated (crooked) septum (the *septum* is the bony cartilage between your nostrils), it can block one of both sides of your nose, leading to a runny or congested nose. Because the resulting symptoms resemble allergic rhinitis, examination of your septum should be part of your physical examination. Surgical correction of a deviated septum may be necessary to relieve severe nasal airway obstruction.

TELLTALE SIGNS: SALUTES, SHINERS, AND CREASES

The symptoms of allergic rhinitis that we list in this chapter often produce a distinctive combination of gestures and facial features, particularly in children and adolescents. If you or someone close to you seems to suffer from allergic rhinitis, keep these sufferer-specific characteristics in mind. These physical signs are often so distinctive that physicians can usually tell, when looking in the waiting room, who are the likely allergic rhinitis sufferers. When my children were younger, I noticed similar traits among the children's friends who had allergies as well. The following gestures and facial formations are characteristics that you and your doctor should look for to help diagnose your specific condition:

- **Allergic salute:** As tempting as if might be consider this gesture as a sign of respect for your physician, the allergic salute actually describes the way that most people use the palm of their hand to rub and raise the tip of their nose to relieve nasal itching and congestion (and possibly to wipe away some mucus).

- **Allergic shiner:** Allergic rhinitis symptoms can really beat up some patients. Dark circles under the eyes due to the swelling and discoloration caused by congestion of small blood vessels beneath the skin in this area can give you the appearance of having gone a few rounds with the heavy weight champion of the world.

- **Allergic (adenoidal) face:** Allergic rhinitis may cause swelling of the *adenoids* (lymph tissue that lines the back of the throat and extends behind the nose), resulting in a sort of tired and droopy appearance.

- **Nasal crease:** This line across the bridge of the nose is usually the result — particularly in children — of rubbing the nose (allergic salute) to relieve nasal congestion and itching.

- **Mouth breathing:** Cases of allergic rhinitis in which severe nasal congestion occurs can result in chronic mouth breathing, leading to the development of a high, arched palate, an elevated upper lip, and an overbite. (This symptom is one of the many reasons why so many teens with allergic rhinitis wind up at the orthodontist.)

The eyes have it: Allergic conjunctivitis

Symptoms such as redness over your eyeballs and the underside of your eyelids, as well as swollen, itchy, and tearing eyes, are characteristic of what doctors refer to as *allergic rhinoconjunctivitis.* This ailment often coexists with allergic rhinitis, and most of the same allergens as those involved with allergic rhinitis can trigger season or perennial outbreaks of this conjunctivitis.

All that drips isn't allergic

Many people think that runny, congested noses and sneezing are always the result of an allergic reaction. However, be aware that rhinitis also comes in nonallergic flavors, such as the following types:

>> **Vasomotor:** The most typical examples of this form of nonallergic rhinitis are the nasal congestion, runny nose, and sneezing that can occur as a result of sudden temperature changes (for example, a blast of cold air). Exposure to bright lights, or irritants, such as tobacco smoke, perfume, bleach, paint fumes, newsprint, automotive emissions, and solvents can also trigger vasomotor rhinitis.

>> **Idiopathic chronic nonallergic rhinitis:** The symptoms are like those of allergic rhinitis but allergies don't cause it. The symptoms include sneezing, stuffy, drippy nose, and mucus in the throat and cough. It's often a long-term problem where now clear cause can be identified. The factors that trigger symptoms can vary from person to person and can include dust, fumes, irritants in the air, and even hot or spicy foods (known as *gustatory rhinitis*). This condition is referred to interchangeably with vasomotor rhinitis by many patients and physicians. In addition, there are some forms of nonallergic rhinitis where eosinophils are found in the nasal secretions (NARES) and are often more receptive to treatment with intranasal steroids.

>> **Infectious:** Upper-respiratory viral ailments such as the common cold are often the cause of acute or chronic nasal distress.

>> **Hormonal:** Women may experience severe nasal congestion while taking birth control pills, as well as during ovulation or during pregnancy — most notably from the second month to the full term. In pregnancy cases, congested nose symptoms usually disappear after delivery.

>> **Emotional:** Men and women may experience runny and congested noses during sexual arousal. Other intensely emotional situations (such as laughing or crying) can also provoke your nose to run or congest.

>> **Atrophic rhinitis:** This form of rhinitis occurs when there's nasal dryness and the tissue inside your nose thins or atrophies. This condition causes chronic nasal dryness and crusting. It's often seen in older patients.

Table 4-1 classifies the different types of allergic and nonallergic rhinitis and lists the main causes of each type.

TABLE 4-1   **Main Causes of Allergic and Nonallergic Rhinitis**

Allergic Rhinitis		Nonallergic Rhinitis	
Type	Causes	Type	Causes
Seasonal (hay fever)	Pollen from trees, grasses, and ragweed	Vasomotor rhinitis	Temperature changes, strong odors, and humidity.
Perennial	Year-round allergens including dust mites, mold, animal dander, cigarette smoke	Idiopathic chronic nonallergic rhinitis	Several triggers, including weather and temperature fluctuations, air pollution, hormonal changes and stress. Exact cause is unknown.
Occupational	Workplace allergens, lab animals, wood, dust, latex	Infectious rhinitis	Viral or bacterial infections (for example, common cold).
		Drug-induced rhinitis	Medications (for example, NSAIDs, ACE inhibitors).
		Hormonal rhinitis	Pregnancy or other hormonal changes.
		Gustatory rhinitis	Hot and/or spicy foods.
		Atrophic rhinitis	Aging, heredity, infections, nutritional deficiencies.
		Nonallergic rhinitis with eosinophilia syndrome (NARES)	Eosinophil infiltration without allergic sensitization.

SEE YOUR DOCTOR

In order to effectively diagnose your condition, a physician must review your medical history, as well as your family's history of allergies, and perform a physical examination. If your family physician suspects a form of allergic rhinitis, they'll probably refer you to specialist, such as an allergist (someone like Dr. Berger) or an otolaryngologist (an ear, nose, and throat doctor), in the following situations:

>> If clarification and identification of the triggers of your condition are needed.

>> If the management of your allergic or nonallergic rhinitis isn't resulting in a substantial improvement of your condition, due to inadequate treatment and/or adverse reactions to medications.

>> If you need to learn how to avoid allergens and irritants that may be triggering your symptoms (see Chapter 5).

>> If your rhinitis or side effects of medications of the condition impair your abilities to perform in your career or occupation (especially in operating an airplane or motor vehicle).

>> If the disease has a significant adverse effect on your quality of life by affecting your comfort or well-being.

>> If rhinitis complications develop, such as sinusitis, *otitis* (ear inflammation), and facial signs (see the "Telltale signs: Salutes, shiners, and creases" sidebar in this chapter).

>> If you have coexisting conditions such as recurring or chronic sinusitis (see Chapter 7), asthma (see Chapter 8) or other respiratory condition, otitis (see Chapter 7), or nasal polyps.

>> If your physician needs to prescribe oral (systemic) corticosteroids (see Chapter 6) to control symptoms.

>> If your symptoms last more than three months.

>> If your medications costs are a financial hardship.

SEE YOUR DOCTOR

In addition to performing a general observation to check for allergic salute, allergic shiners, allergic face, mouth breathing, and facial pallor (a pale face is often a sign of fatigue), your physician will examine the following areas:

>> The front of your nose to check for an allergic crease and the condition of your septum (the "great divide" of cartilage between your nostrils).

>> Your nasal passages, to check for swelling of the nasal turbinates (protruding tissues that line the interior of the nose — see Figure 4-1), nasal polyps (pale, round or pear-shaped, smooth, gelatinous outgrowths of the nasal lining), congestion, and the character, color, and amount of secretions from your nose.

>> The inside of your mouth and the back of your throat for redness, swelling, enlarges or diseased tonsils, and to check drainage from the nasal cavity. In addition, your physician may check for the presence of a high arched palate and/or *malocclusion* (misalignment of jaw and teeth, due to mouth breathing and tongue thrusting).

>> Your neck and face, for lumps and sensitive, painful, or numb areas.

>> Your eyes and ears, for signs of inflammation and/or infection.

>> If indicated, further examination might include checking your vocal cords, adenoids, sinuses, and *Eustachian tubes* (the connection between your middle ear, nose, and throat that causes your ears to pop when descending in an airplane).

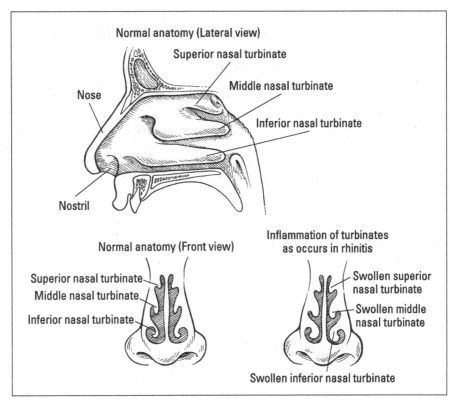

FIGURE 4-1: The two cross-sections show the difference between a healthy nose and one with rhinitis.

In addition to evaluating your physiological condition, your physician also attempts to determine

>> The pattern, frequency, and seasonal variations of the allergic reactions that you experience.

>> The types of allergens and irritants to which you may be exposed at home, work, school, friends' and relative's homes, and other locations that you frequent, such as malls, theaters, restaurants — even modes of transport, such as vehicles, trains, boats, and airplanes.

SKIN TESTS: THE GOLD STANDARD

Your physician may also need to conduct allergy skin tests to confirm and identify the specific allergens that trigger your condition. In some cases, skin testing can also indicate your level of sensitivity to the allergens that bother you. A skin test procedure generally involves the physician placing a drop of a suspected allergen on your skin and then using a device that pricks, punctures, or scratches the area to see whether the allergen produces a reaction. If you're allergic to that specific allergen, your skin reacts in a way that resembles a mosquito bite or hive. If you're on pins and needles to gather more information about skin tests, see Chapter 3.

Managing Rhinitis

Three basic approaches exist for treating and managing allergies, including forms of allergic rhinitis.

Avoidance

Benjamin Franklin once advised, "An ounce of prevention is worth a pound of cure." Eliminating (or at least lessening) your exposure to allergens and irritants can often result in less severe symptoms and less need for medication. In Chapter 5, we give you more detailed advice on what allergens and irritants to avoid and how to avoid them, especially in your home and bedroom, where most people spend the greater parts of their lives.

Pharmacotherapy

Pharmacotherapy is the term physicians use for treating patients with medications. This form of therapy is particularly important in allergic disease, because complete avoidance of allergens can be difficult. Therefore, your physician may also recommend or prescribe one of more medications to help manage your condition, depending on the nature and severity of your symptoms, occupation, age, and other factors that your physician may assess. We provide and in-depth analysis of these products and their recommended uses and side effects in Chapter 6.

Immunotherapy

If your physician concludes that avoidance and drug therapies don't provide effective results, and if the severity of your symptoms or the nature of your occupation warrants it, they may advise you to consider *immunotherapy*, otherwise known as *desensitization, hyposensitization*, or just plain-old *allergy shots*. Immunotherapy treatment for allergic rhinitis generally requires at least three years of injections. (For an in-depth discussion of immunotherapy, turn to Chapter 6.)

Considering special cases

Certain groups of patients with allergic rhinitis require more specialized treatment and consideration. These groups include

>> **Children:** Intranasal corticosteroid sprays are often recommended as the first line of treatment in children with allergic rhinitis as they have been shown to be very safe and effective, even for long-term use. Your physician may also prescribe an oral antihistamine to manage your child's symptoms. Oral decongestants such as pseudoephedrine (Sudafed) are considered to be safe for older children (older than 6 years); however, they should only be used under strict medical supervision, in children younger than 4 years old.

>> **Elderly people:** Doctors generally advise that elderly patients use nonsedating antihistamines, which produce fewer significant side effects, instead of sedating antihistamine products, such as diphenhydramine (Benadryl). In addition, topical nasal corticosteroids can often be recommended for elderly patients.

SEE YOUR DOCTOR

>> **Pregnant women:** Physicians often recommend nasal saline irrigation as a first line treatment option for the management of allergic rhinitis symptoms in pregnant women. Oral antihistamines (Cetirizine) are also considered to be a safe and effective option. Recent guidelines recommend that oral decongestants should be avoided during the first trimester of pregnancy, but your physician may prescribe nasal decongestant sprays (Afrin, Neo-Synephrine) and topic nasal corticosteroids (Flonase) for short-term relief from the second trimester onwards. Always consult your physician before starting any new medication while pregnant (see Dr. Berger's book *Asthma For Dummies* for more information on this topic.)

REMEMBER

>> **Athletes:** Your physician needs to make sure that any recommended OTC or prescription product isn't on any sports federation's list of banned substances. The U.S. Olympic Committee (USOC) and the International Olympic Committee ban the use of all oral and topical nasal decongestants and oral corticosteroids. In addition, some international sports federations also ban the use of oral antihistamines. Using other nasal products may require written approval by governing sports bodies.

WORRIED ABOUT WORSENING HAY FEVER . . . IT'S NOT ALL IN YOUR HEAD!!

If you notice your allergic rhinitis symptoms appear to be getting worse and are lasting longer in recent years, climate change may be to blame! There are several reasons for this:

- **Extended pollen seasons:** Rising temperatures extend the growing seasons of many allergenic plants, prolonging the period of pollen release by as much as 30 days.

- **Increased pollen production:** Elevated atmospheric carbon dioxide (CO_2) levels act as a stimulant for plant growth and pollen production.

- **Air pollution and allergen sensitivity:** Climate change contributes to increased air pollution, which compromises respiratory tract defenses. This heightened sensitivity may make allergic rhinitis sufferers more susceptible to the inflammatory effects of aeroallergens, including pollens.

These factors collectively contribute to more persistent allergen exposure and a worsening of allergic rhinitis symptoms for many sufferers.

Chapter **5**

Avoiding Environmental Allergens

The three main ways of treating allergies are avoidance, pharmacotherapy (treatment with medications), and immunotherapy (treatment that modifies your immune response to allergens). Of these three methods, avoidance, which this chapter discusses, is the most practical and effective tool in most cases.

Avoiding, or at least significantly decreasing, exposure to the substances in your environment that trigger your allergic reactions can often help relieve your symptoms, thus improving your overall health. These avoidance measures can also reduce the need for medication or shots, thereby saving you much time and money.

Explaining Why Avoidance Matters

You've probably heard the joke about the patient who complains, "Doc, it hurts when I do this," to which the doctor replies, "Then stop doing that." Silly as that joke seems, the doctor's advice exemplifies the basic concept of avoidance, whether you're dealing with *allergic rhinitis* (hay fever), *urticaria* (hives), food allergies, other allergies, or asthma. Depending on your sensitivity, avoiding the substance(s) or levels of exposure to the substance(s) that trigger (that's why such substances are called *triggers*) your allergic reaction is critical to effectively manage your symptoms.

In theory, avoidance may seem simple enough. In real life however, the trick is to figure out — short of living in a bubble — the practical and effective steps you can take to minimize your contact with allergy triggers. The following sections explore how to identify your allergy triggers and recognize when you're most at risk. We also describe the steps you can take to avoid being exposed to your allergy triggers in the first place.

Using an avoidance checklist

Environmental control measures are vital components of any allergist's treatment plan. Every practicing allergist focuses on helping you create and implement an effective avoidance strategy for yourself or your partner, child, or other family member, with allergies or asthma who lives with you. The plan that you and your allergist develop will likely include these steps:

1. **Identify allergy triggers in your environment, especially indoor allergens and irritants.**
2. **Recognize situations in which you may come into contact with those allergy triggers.**
3. **Discover how you can avoid allergens or minimize your contact with them.**
4. **Allergy-proof your home.**

Understanding key terminology

In case you're also allergic to jargon, the following list explains the most common technical terms that allergists use when discussing avoidance and allergy-proofing:

>> **Allergen load:** Your total level of exposure, at any one time, to any single allergen or combination of allergens, that trigger your allergies.

>> **Allergic threshold:** Your level of sensitivity to an allergen. A low allergic threshold means that your sensitivity to an allergen is high; even a small exposure to the substance can trigger your symptoms. A high allergic threshold means that your body requires a higher concentration of allergens to trigger symptoms. Your threshold level, however, can decrease if you're exposed too often to large quantities of an allergen or to a combination of allergens.

>> **Allergy trigger:** A normally harmless substance, such as pollen, dust, animal dander, insect stings, and certain foods and drugs, that can provoke an abnormal response by your immune system if you're sensitized to that substance. Physicians usually refer to these substances as *allergens*.

>> **Cross-reactivity:** Your immune system is an expert at recognizing related allergens in seemingly unrelated sources. If you're exposed to these allergen cousins at the same time, your allergen load can exceed your allergic threshold, thereby triggering allergic symptoms.

>> **Desensitization:** In the context of avoidance and allergy proofing, *desensitizing* describes the active process of removing, shielding, or reducing the source of allergens in your environment. Your allergist may advise you to desensitize your home, focusing especially on the bedroom of any person with allergies or asthma. Desensitization is also used to refer the form of treatment in which an allergist injects small amounts of an allergen extract under your skin (called *subcutaneous immunotherapy* (SCIT), or administers allergen orally (oral immunotherapy [OIT] /oral mucosal immunotherapy [OMIT]) so your body can gradually "learns" not to react to the substance (see Chapter 4).

>> **HEPA:** High Efficiency Particulate Air. An air filtration process developed for hospital operating rooms and other locations requires a sterilized environment. HEPA filters absorb and contain 99.97 percent of all particles larger than 0.3 microns (one three-hundredth the width of a human hair). If the unit truly operates at that level, only 3 out of 10,000 particles manage to sneak back into the room. Vacuum cleaners and air purifiers with ULPA (see definition later in this list) and HEPA filters are a vital tool for desensitizing and allergy-proofing your indoor environment.

>> **HVAC:** Heating, ventilation, and air-conditioning systems are your home's lungs. The quality of air that you breathe indoors is largely dependent on the condition of these systems and the air that flows into and out of your environment through them.

>> **ULPA:** Ultra Low Penetration Air. Even more thorough than the HEPA process, this filtration system is designed to absorb and contain 99.99 percent of all particles larger than 0.12 microns.

Knowing your limits

Avoidance measures rarely require the complete elimination of all allergy triggers and irritants in your environment. In many cases, you may only need to limit your exposure to certain triggers in order to prevent or alleviate symptoms.

REMEMBER

Think of your allergic threshold as a cup and the allergy triggers in your environment as liquid pouring into that cup. Overflowing your small cup (low allergic threshold) may require only a small amount of liquid (allergens), thereby triggering an allergic reaction. A larger cup — a higher threshold — can accommodate more liquid without overflowing (without triggering an allergic reaction). The key to mastering your threshold is knowing your limit.

Another important concept to keep in mind when considering avoidance is to imagine a balance or scale with your allergic threshold on one side and your allergen load on the other. You won't set off your allergies unless the level of exposure to allergen triggers overloads your allergic threshold. Keep in mind, however, that your scales can tip, not only from excessive exposure to a single allergen, but also from exposure to small amounts of a variety of allergens which can increase the total allergen load.

Cross-reactivity: Pollen food allergy syndrome/oral allergy syndrome

Cross-reactivity is also an important factor in causing allergic reactions, and it can contribute to overloading your allergic threshold. For example, if you have a sensitivity to ragweed, you may also have a sensitivity to allergens in melons such as honeydew, cantaloupe, and watermelon. In fact, up to 75 percent of adults allergic to birch tree pollen (a springtime pollen) can experience mouth or throat symptoms after eating apples, celery, or peanuts. It turns out that food allergens that produce oral allergy reactions are easily degraded by heat and stomach acid. As a result, when these allergens reach the stomach with its highly acidic environment, they're destroyed and therefore don't produce systemic allergic reactions, but only local reactions in the oral cavity.

This phenomenon occurs because in some individuals, an allergenic cross-reactivity exists between certain food proteins and nonfood protein sources that can look similar to immune systems. As a result, during ragweed season — in addition to ragweed allergy symptoms — you might also experience itching and swelling of your mouth and lips when eating melons, even though these fruits may not present a problem for you during the rest of the year. Some people also experience cross-reactivity reactions between latex (see Chapter 12) and bananas, avocados, papaya, kiwi, and chestnuts.

Pollen food allergy syndrome (PFAS), also called oral allergy syndrome (OAS), is linked to seasonal pollen allergies and can mimic an allergic reaction to the food; however, symptoms tend to be mild, transient, and restricted to the oral cavity.

TIP

Avoid eating these raw foods especially during pollen allergy season (trees in spring, ragweed in the fall), because frequently PFAS worsens during the particular pollen season. Sometimes baking the food or peeling it before eating (for example, apples) can reduce the cross reaction of the food because high temperature breaks down the proteins associated with PFAS, and in some cases, those allergenic proteins can be concentrated on the skin of the fruit.

Targeting Allergens in the Home

Early on, our ancestors realized that getting out of the elements and into some type of shelter was a key aspect of surviving the dangers and challenges of the prehistoric world. For the most part, humans have become indoor creatures, progressing from cave and tree dwellings to suburbs, malls, and tightly sealed office buildings. In dwellings, humans are safe (for the most part) from predators (being safe from other humans is another story), and most people possess the means to shield themselves from the adversities of weather and climate.

One of the downsides of modern structures is that indoor environments, at home, work, and school, and even in cars and other enclosed means of transportation, can often contain far more significant sources of triggers than outdoor environments. Most enclosures concentrate irritants and allergens, and because people spend so much of their time indoors, that's where people often experience significant exposure to allergy triggers.

Energy-conservation building codes adopted in the United States since the 1970s have worsened the concentration of allergens in structures, because airborne particles that contain allergens, as well as irritants, can often remain trapped indoors. So, although we're certainly in favor of energy efficient structures, you need to ensure that the air you breathe inside — especially at home — is as safe as possible.

Indoor allergens

If you have allergic rhinitis, you may be focusing your attention solely on pollen counts, air pollution, and other elements of the outdoor environment as the prime sources for allergens and irritants that trigger your symptoms. You may have also assumed that indoor air is cleaner and safer than the air that you breathe outside. However, according to Environmental Protection Agency (EPA) studies, indoor air can contain as much as 70 times the pollution of outdoor air.

According to the American Lung Association, most Americans spend 90 percent of their time indoors and 60 percent of that time is at home. Therefore, indoor air pollution is a serious concern, particularly because studies show that it can cause or aggravate allergies and asthma.

Allergens on the barbie?

The issue of outdoor and indoor exposure to allergens and irritants is analogous to the difference between barbecuing outside or inside. When you cook outside, the smoke dissipates. This backyard barbecue process is similar to the way outdoor air dilutes the effects of pollutants and allergens.

If you were crazy enough to bring your grill inside, seal all the windows and doors, turn off the ventilation, and then fire up the coals, within two minutes smoke would fill your house. Now, imagine indoor allergens and irritants as that smoke. All too frequently, many people breathe this polluted air in their indoor environments. The allergy-proofing steps that we discuss in this chapter show you how to avoid and control this type of indoor air pollution.

Allergy-Proofing Your Home

TIP

Allergen avoidance begins at home. While we certainly advise you to avoid or limit exposure to allergens and irritants outside — as well as at work, school, or other indoor locations — avoidance therapy can actually have the most beneficial impact in your home. Even if you're exposed to allergy triggers outside your home, reducing your exposure to those allergens and irritants at home may prevent your allergen threshold from overflowing or overloading.

On average, most people spend one-third of their lives in the bedroom — much of that time in bed. Hence, your bedroom is the most important single area in your home. After you allergy-proof your bedroom, try to use it as much as possible to insure that you can give your allergies a rest.

In and around the home the most common and important sources of allergens that you should focus on when you're allergy-proofing are

>> Dust and dust mites

>> Pets

>> Mold

>> Pollen

Controlling irritants at home is also vital to successful avoidance therapy. Although these substances don't trigger an allergic response by your body's immune system — as is the case with allergens — they often worsen existing allergy or asthma conditions.

Tobacco smoke is the most significant irritant found in the home that aggravates allergy and asthma reactions. Other important irritants, in alphabetical order, include the following:

>> Aerosols, paints, and smoke from wood-burning stoves

>> Glue

>> Household cleaners

>> Perfumes and scents

>> Scented soaps

Figure 5-1 illustrates the basics of allergy-proofing, which we detail in the following sections.

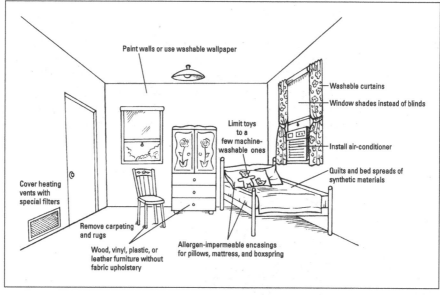

FIGURE 5-1: An allergy-proofed bedroom.

© John Wiley & Sons, Inc.

Controlling the dust in your house

House dust is one of the most prevalent allergy triggers in any home, and unfortunately, it's everywhere. Think of house dust as one of life's inevitabilities — along with death and taxes. House dust can trigger allergy symptoms either as an irritant to sensitized target organs (such as your eyes, nose, or lungs) or as a result of the specific allergens often contained in house dust.

Studies show that the average six-room home in the U.S. collects 40 pounds of dust each year. Please note, however, that dust is not dirt, nor is it an indication of poor housekeeping. House dust is a normal breakdown product of fibers found in pillows, drapes, clothes, linens, and other furnishings at home, work, school, or even in your car.

Ridding your house of dust mites

Allergy-proofing your bedroom and home likely involves dealing with dust mites more than with any other allergy trigger, because these microscopic creatures produce the single largest component of house dust that triggers allergies. Eighty percent of patients with allergies test positive for sensitivity to the dust mite allergen. The dust mite allergen is also the most significant allergic trigger of asthma attacks.

The most potent allergen in house dust comes from the house dust mite (*dermatophagoides pteronyssinus* and/or *dermatophagoides farinae*, depending on where you live). Check out Figure 5-2 to see a dust mite. These tiny, eight-legged microscopic spider relatives live in dust where they feed on dead skin flakes that warm blooded creatures in house such as humans, constantly shed (hence the scientific name *dermatophagoides*, meaning skin-eater; but don't worry — dust mites don't eat living skin) at rates of up to 1.5 grams per clay — that's a lot of dust mite chow.

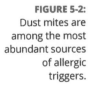

FIGURE 5-2:
Dust mites are among the most abundant sources of allergic triggers.

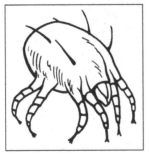

©John Wiley & Sons, Inc.

Because dust mites usually are as snug as bugs in a rug, people rarely come into direct contact with the live creatures themselves — just with their waste or decomposing bodies, which also can be a significant source of house dust allergens. So, although you've probably never seen them, dust mites are a fact of life — they're bound to follow almost anyplace you settle.

Controlling dust mites in the bedroom

Few people ever go to bed alone. Dust mites thrive in dark and humid environments such as mattresses, pillows, and box springs. In fact, the average bed contains two million dust mites, which means that you may breathe in significant amounts of dust mite allergens while you sleep. Dust mites also survive well in blankets, carpets, towels, upholstered furniture, drapery, and children's stuffed toys.

Although eradication of these natural inhabitants of your home is virtually impossible — the females lay 20 to 50 eggs every three weeks — you can take practical and effective steps to minimize exposure to dust mite allergens.

TIP

In our experience, taking the following measures often results in a significant decrease in allergic symptoms and medication requirements for patients with allergies or asthma:

>> **Beds:** Encase all pillows, mattresses, and box springs in special allergen impermeable encasings, and mount all beds on bed frames. Wash all bed linens in hot water (at least 130 degrees) every two weeks. Only use pillows, blankets, quilts, and bedspreads made of synthetic materials. Avoid down- (feather) filled comforters and pillows.

>> **Climate control:** Don't locate your bedroom in a humid area such as the basement. Likewise, use an air conditioner or dehumidifier to keep the humidity in your home below 50 percent. You may want to use a humidity gauge to monitor humidity levels.

>> **Carpets and drapes:** If possible, go for the bare look in your home — remove carpeting and thick rugs. Bare surfaces such as hard wood, linoleum, or tile are inhospitable to dust mites and are also much easier to clean, thereby minimizing dust buildup. If you can't remove your carpeting and rugs, treat them with products that inactivate dust mite allergens. We also recommend washable curtains or window shades rather than heavy drapery or blinds.

>> **Housekeeping:** Vacuum thoroughly, at least once a week, with a HEPA or ULPA vacuum cleaner (see the section "Understanding key terminology" earlier in this chapter). If you have allergies, wear a dust mask when you clean or engage in any activity that stirs up dust. Also, consider cleaning your furniture with a tannic acid solution.

- **Ventilation:** Use HEPA air cleaners to keep the indoor air throughout your home as pure as possible. (Refer to the section "Understanding key terminology" earlier in this chapter.) Cover any heating vents with special vent filters to clean the air before it enters your rooms. Install a room HEPA or ULPA filter in the bedroom and run it 24/7 while keeping the bedroom door closed. Be sure to buy a filter with specs that cover the size of the room under filtration.

- **Decorations and furnishings:** Use furniture made of wood, vinyl, plastic, and leather throughout your home instead of furniture made of upholstery. Likewise, make your bedroom as uncluttered and wipeable as possible. Avoid shelves, pennants, posters, photos or pictures, heavy cushions, and other dust collectors. Limit the clothes, books, and other personal objects in your bedroom to the essentials, and make sure that you shut closets or drawers when not in use.

REMEMBER

If your child has allergies or asthma, don't make their bedroom a stuffed animal zoo; try to limit those types of toys to a few machine washable ones. Keep your child's stuffed animals and toys in the closet or in a closed chest, container, or drawer when not in use.

Regulating pet dander

Pets are cherished members of many households. However, dander (skin flakes) from these animals is a significant source of allergy triggers for many people. All warm-blooded household pets, regardless of hair length, produce proteins in their dander and saliva that can trigger allergies. Dead skin cells in their dander can even serve as a food supply for dust mites. Cat dander residue can linger at significant exposure levels in carpets for up to 20 weeks and in mattresses for years, even after you remove the animal.

REMEMBER

We usually advise people with allergies or asthma not to introduce a new pet into their home. If you already have a pet, we realize that removing this family member can be a very emotional issue for you and other household members, even though Fluffy or Fido's dander may be triggering your allergies or those of your children.

TIP

If finding a new home for your pet isn't likely, we advise the following measures:

- Keep your pet outdoors whenever possible.

- If keeping your pet outdoors isn't possible, by all means, keep the pet out of the patient's bedroom.

- Make sure that anyone who touches your pet washes their hands before contacting the patient or entering the patient's bedroom.

>> Washing your pet with water once a week may remove surface allergens and possibly reduce the amount of dander that can stick to other household members' clothes and body (thereby reaching the patient's bedroom). Although it may take some training (and a few scratch marks), even cats can get used to baths.

Controlling mold in your abode

Molds are some of the oldest and most common organisms on the planet, and they're widespread in most homes. Think of molds as microscopic fungi or mushrooms. You've probably encountered various forms of mold at home, from splotches on your shower door to the greenish growth on that tomato you forgot at the back of your fridge last year (hope your mom doesn't find out).

Molds release fungal spores into the air, which settle on organic matter and grow into new mold clusters. When inhaled by sensitized individuals, these airborne spores can trigger allergic symptoms. Airborne mold spores are more numerous than pollen grains, and unlike pollen, they don't have a limited season. In many parts of the United States and Canada, mold spores may be present until the first snow cover.

Outdoor molds can enter your home through the air, by blowing in open windows and doors, and through vents. Indoor molds can grow year-round, and they thrive in dark, humid areas of the home, such as basements and bathrooms. Molds also grow under carpets, and in pillows, mattresses, air conditioners, garbage containers, and refrigerators. The older your home, the larger the amount of mold that grows there.

TIP

Limiting your exposure to mold spores is a key part of allergy-proofing your home. We advise the following steps for controlling molds in and around your home:

>> Avoid damp areas of your home, such as an unfinished basement or a room with a water leak. Or use a dehumidifier to lower humidity in those areas to 35 to 40 percent.

>> Make sure your clothes dryer vents to the outside.

>> Ventilate your bathroom well, especially after a shower or bath. Use mold-killing and mold-preventing solutions behind the toilet and around the sink, shower, bathtub, washing machine, refrigerator, and other areas of your home where water or moisture collects.

>> Clean any visible mold from the walls, floors, and ceiling by using a nonchlorine bleach.

>> Take out the trash and clean your garbage container regularly to prevent mold growth.

>> Dry out damp footwear and clothing in which mold could breed. Don't hang clothes outside, where they can become landing areas for mold spores.

>> Limit the number of indoor plants or remove them altogether, because mold may grow in potting soil. Dried flowers may also contain mold, so avoid them.

TIP

If you have allergies or asthma, avoid exposure to outdoor molds around your home. These molds proliferate in fallen leaves, compost, cut grass, fertilizer hay, and barns. If you need to work in your yard, wear a well-fitting face mask. Cut back any heavy vegetation around your home to allow the structure to breathe and to prevent dampness and mold growth.

Pollen-proofing

Pollens can trigger allergic rhinitis and asthma symptoms. Allergic rhinitis is perhaps the best-known allergy of all. Many people associate this type of allergy primarily with outdoor exposure to pollen. However, you may also experience significant levels of pollen at home, and these exposures can also trigger allergic rhinitis symptoms.

Most pollens are windborne, and they can often blow indoors (typically through open windows and doors) and trigger allergic symptoms such as allergic rhinitis within your home, not just outdoors. Wind-pollinated trees, grasses, and weeds produce pollen during various times of the year.

These plants release their pollens in huge quantities to reproduce. For example, ragweed plants may release up to 1 million pollen granules in a day, and the massive amounts of pollen granules that some trees release, can resemble clouds.

Pollens are such universal features of life on the planet that pollen samples from excavation sites enable archaeologists and botanists to reconstruct what the natural environments of ancient times probably were like.

TIP

Take the following steps, especially during periods of high pollination, to avoid excessive exposure to pollen:

>> Avoid intense outdoor activities, such as exercise or strenuous work, during the early morning and late afternoon hours when pollen counts are highest. If you need to work outside, wear a pollen and dust mask.

>> Close windows and run a HEPA or ULPA air conditioner and air purifier.

>> Make sure to clean and replace your air conditioner filters regularly.

>> Wash your hair before going to bed to avoid getting pollen on your pillow.

>> Use a clothes dryer instead of hanging the wash outside, where it acts as a filter trap for pollen. You may like the idea of fresh, air-dried laundry, but your target organs (see Chapter 4) won't enjoy the allergic reactions that all the fresh pollen triggers, especially if you hang sheets and pillowcases out on the line.

Focusing on more pollen particulars

Seed-bearing plants reproduce by pollination, which involves the transfer of pollen granules — the plants' sperm cells — from male parts of a plant to receptive female reproductive sites. When pollen granules reach female sites, they produce pollen tubes that carry the sperm cells close to the female reproductive cells. (See, technical stuff can sometimes be exciting!)

A variety of means, including insects, animals, and the wind, provide transportation for pollen granules. Windborne pollens that trigger allergic rhinitis symptoms come from three classifications of plants:

>> **Grasses:** The grasses that cause most grass-induced allergic rhinitis are widespread throughout North America and were imported from Europe to feed animals and create lawns. By contrast, the many native grasses of North America produce little pollen.

>> **Weeds:** The most important weeds that trigger symptoms of allergic rhinitis are those of the tribe Ambrosieae, known as ragweeds.

>> **Trees:** Most trees that release symptom-causing pollens are angiosperms (which means "flowering seeds," and yet these trees don't actually flower), such as willows, poplars, beeches, or oaks. Similarly, pollen from a few gymnosperms (naked seeds), such as pines, spruces, firs, junipers, cypresses, hemlocks, and cedars, also can trigger symptom of allergic rhinitis.

Although these plant groups account for most cases of pollen-induced allergic rhinitis, only a small percentage of the members of each group has been shown to produce allergenic pollen.

Blowing in the wind

Wind pollination has worked well for certain plants for millions of years, enabling many of them to survive and flourish in environments that don't provide many insect or animal pollinators. The much younger species of man (Homo sapiens — us) has also flourished in these areas, with the result that you're often in the pollen path of wind-pollinating plants. Instead of windborne pollen granules reaching their intended targets, they often end up in your eyes, nose, throat, and lungs, causing allergic reactions in susceptible individuals.

Recognizing pollens (and molds) for all seasons

Most wind-pollinating plants in the United States and Canada release their pollens at specific times during the year that can be classified into five pollen seasons. Whenever your respiratory symptoms begin or worsen during one of these seasons, the predominance of specific pollens during that particular time of year may be the cause of the allergic reactions that complicate your asthma.

Here's the type of pollen (or molds) that may affect you in each of the five pollen seasons:

>> When your symptoms get worse during spring, the probable cause is tree pollen.

>> In late spring and early summer, grass pollen is the likely culprit.

>> From late summer to autumn, weed pollen, especially from ragweed, may cause you problems.

>> Especially during the summer and fall but also throughout the year except during snow cover — mold spores, particularly those of airborne molds — may trigger your allergies.

>> In winter, windborne pollens rarely are a factor in most parts of the United States and Canada. However, in the warmer southern regions of the United States that don't experience prolonged periods of freezing temperatures (such as southern California), pollinating plants and molds still release allergy-triggering pollen and mold spores whenever there's no snow cover.

When your allergic rhinitis symptoms follow a seasonal pattern, consult your physician to find out whether specific pollens are the problem. You may also want to ask them for information on the major aeroallergens for the area 50 to 100 miles around where you live and work.

Including the effect of nonnatives

A list of local allergenic plants can serve as a good starting point for figuring out what plants may be affecting your allergies. However, knowing about nonnative plants in your environment is also useful.

Nonnative plants in your environment often include trees and grasses — some of which may also produce allergenic pollen — that may have been planted around your community for decorative purposes.

RAGWEED TO STARBOARD CAPTAIN!

Is that seasickness or allergies? Ragweed pollen has such a broad range that it has been detected 400 miles out to sea. So, if you're on the ocean during ragweed season, we suggest taking, your medication with you. (Make sure it's not drowsy, especially when you're the helm!)

Counting your pollens

Many newspapers, television, online weather sites, and radio news programs regularly report pollen counts. The pollen count is the measurement of the total number of granules of a particular kind of pollen per cubic meter of air per day.

Pollen counters rate the resulting numbers according to five categories, ranging from absent to very high.

Running the numbers

Bear in mind that the severity of symptoms triggered by pollens depends, not only on the actual pollen count, but also on the particular pollen being measured. In addition, the proximity of the collection station to the particular pollen being reported usually affects the actual count; moreover, each region of the world has its own predominant allergy-producing pollens. Table 5-1 provides the generally accepted guidelines for interpreting pollen counts for ragweed, which is the most closely followed type of pollen count in many parts of the United States and Canada.

TABLE 5-1   **Ragweed Pollen Count Guidelines**

Category	Pollen Grains Per Cubic Meter Per Day*	Degree of Symptoms
Absent	0	No symptoms.
Low	0-10	Symptoms may only affect people with extreme sensitivities to these pollens.
Moderate	0-50	Many people who are sensitive to these pollens experience symptoms at this rating.
High	50-500	Most people with any sensitivity to these pollens experience symptoms.
Very High	More than 500	Almost anyone with any sensitivity at all to these pollens experiences symptoms. If you're extremely sensitive to ragweed pollen, your symptoms can be severe at this level.

These figures are averages

TAKE MY POLLEN PLEASE!

Plants that are the main culprits in allergic rhinitis depend on wind pollination because they're not pretty or colorful enough to attract insects or other animals to do the pollinating. Most flowers that appeal to people — and to insects and other animals — produce heavier pollens that stick to the insects or animals that carry it to female plant reproductive sites, so you're far less likely to acquire sensitivities to pollen from roses or other attractive, colorful plants, unless you experience constant, close contact with flowers. When you experience allergy symptoms after stopping to smell the roses, pollens from nearby grasses, weeds, or trees may cause your reaction.

Here are some other factors to keep in mind when reading a pollen count.

>> Today's pollen count was collected yesterday and usually reflects what was in the air 24 hours ago.

>> Rain can clear pollen out of the air temporarily. However, short thunderstorms — the kind that are characteristic of late spring and summer in parts of North America — can actually spread pollen granules farther.

>> Hot weather increases pollination, whereas (you probably figured that one out already) cooler temperatures reduce the amount of pollen plants produce.

>> Pollen grains typically are at their highest concentrations from mid-morning to early afternoon.

>> Because they're windborne, many pollen granules travel great distances, so the plants in your backyard or your neighbor's garden may not be triggering your allergies. Chopping down the olive tree in the front of your house may have little, if any, effect on your allergies.

Considering climate change

Climate change is making pollen allergies worse. As the planet warms and more carbon dioxide is released into the atmosphere, scientists are reporting lengthening pollen seasons and increased pollen levels. Warmer winter temperatures are leading to earlier spring pollen seasons lasting later into the fall and more pollen production per plant.

Noting quality not quantity

Not all pollens are equal. Studies show that a little pollen from grasses, such as Bermuda and bluegrass or trees such as oak and elm, can go a long way in triggering allergies. On the other hand, your allergic rhinitis symptoms usually are triggered only by much higher and direct exposures to pine and eucalyptus pollen.

These pollens are large and heavy and don't disperse widely in the wind. Similarly, a moderate ragweed pollen count usually has far more effect than even a high English plantain count, depending especially on your sensitivity to those pollens. So, knowing the types of pollens that are blowing in the wind, and how much of those pollens are actually in the wind, is important.

DOCTOR SAYS

GO WEST YOUNG POLLEN!

When I was a boy growing up in New York, I remember my physician telling patients with asthma to move to Arizona because of the area's dry climate and sparse plant population. Through the years, plenty of folk have indeed moved to Arizona (and not just because of my physician). Many of Arizona's new residents decided to plant nonnative ornamental plants, such as mulberry trees, to spruce up the desert scenery. Mulberry trees thrive in the hot, dry climate and produce clouds of allergenic pollen. As a result, Phoenix and other cities in the state are now major allergy centers. In fact, some of the busiest allergists in the United States practice in Arizona.

DUST GETS IN YOUR EYES ... OR NOSE, THROAT, AND LUNGS

The following is a list of symptoms that you can use to determine whether inhalant allergens in house dust trigger your respiratory symptoms:

- You experience asthma and/or allergy symptoms as a result of dusting, making beds, or changing blankets and bed linens.

- Your symptoms seem to occur year-round rather than seasonally.

- Your symptoms are worse when you're indoors.

- Your symptoms are worse when you awaken in bed in the morning.

Chapter **6**

Treating Your Rhinitis

f you have *allergic rhinitis* (hay fever), you can significantly improve your quality of life by taking avoidance measures and allergy-proofing your home and office, decreasing your exposure to the substances that trigger your allergic reactions and, in most cases, your nasal allergy symptoms. (See Chapter 5 for more on allergy-proofing and avoidance measures.) However, because allergens such as pollens, molds, and dust are everywhere, complete avoidance can be difficult, if not impossible. Fortunately, many types of allergy medications are available. If used properly — based on your physician's advice — medications can prevent or relieve your allergic reactions.

In this chapter, we explain how the most common nasal allergy medications work, the potential side effects of each, and how you can make the best choices to control your allergic reactions. Effectively treating those reactions is often the most important factor in reducing — and, in some cases, even eliminating — many common nasal symptoms, thus improving your overall quality of life.

Getting Familiar with Pharmacology

The many drugs available for treating nasal allergies have various uses and char-acteristics. Some allergy medications are designed for one specific purpose, whereas others have more flexible uses. In general, nasal allergy medications fall into three categories of usage:

>> **Preventive:** If used properly, these types of medications can keep your nasal symptoms from developing. For people who have chronic symptoms of rhinitis, allergic or nonallergic, the most effective approach is to preventively use antihistamines (oral or nasal) and nasal corticosteroid medications (see the "Using nasal corticosteroids" section, later in this chapter).

>> **Stabilizing:** These drugs can often stop a reaction that's already in process before your immune system can release potent chemical mediators of inflammation, such as histamine and leukotrienes, that produce notice-able symptoms.

>> **Relief:** Most of the commonly available over-the-counter (OTC) oral antihista-mines and decongestants fall into this category. Many people use them to relieve the symptoms of rhinitis after symptoms have occurred. As we explain in this chapter, you're usually not taking full advantage of antihistamines and nasal corticosteroid sprays if you only use them after your symptoms have started.

Whether prescribed or purchased OTC, a few basic types of drugs are used to treat nasal allergies, including the following:

>> Antihistamines (available OTC and by prescription in various forms)

>> Antihistamine nasal sprays (available OTC and by prescription)

>> Decongestants (available OTC and by prescription in oral form, or as nonpre-scription nasal sprays and drops)

>> Combinations of antihistamine (available OTC and by prescription in oral form) and decongestant products are also used for multisymptomatic relief, as we discuss in the later section "Two for the Nose: Combination Products"

>> Nasal corticosteroid sprays (available OTC and by prescription)

>> Mast cell stabilizer nasal sprays containing cromolyn (available OTC)

>> *Anticholinergic* (drying) nasal sprays (available only by prescription)

TIP

To get the most out of your treatment, take the time to understand what each medication can do to relieve your symptoms. An informed patient is a healthier patient. If your physician prescribes medication for your allergic rhinitis (or any ailment), don't hesitate to inquire about the product, why it's being prescribed, and any possible side effects.

Blocking Your Histamines: Antihistamines

As the name indicates, *antihistamines* are medications (available in tablet, capsule, liquid, nasal spray form, or injection) that counter the effects of *histamine* — a chemical substance released by the body as the result of injury or in response to an allergen. *First-generation* (sedating) OTC antihistamines have been in use since 1942 and at one time were the first medication option for allergic rhinitis sufferers. We discuss the important differences between first-generation antihistamines and most of the newer *second-generation* (nonsedating or less sedating) antihistamines here.

Both first- and second-generation antihistamines block the effects of histamine and are most effective in controlling or alleviating symptoms such as sneezing, runny nose, and itchy nose, eyes, and throat. However, these medications may not reduce nasal congestion. As a result, they're frequently combined with a decongestant to relieve symptoms of congestion. In addition, antihistamines produce various side effects, depending on the type of product (OTC or prescription), dosage levels, and course of medication.

REMEMBER

If you have asthma, don't be afraid to use antihistamines, depending on your specific condition and your physician's advice. In the past, product information labels advised asthma patients not to use antihistamines because these medications theoretically dry out the airways. However, studies show that the nasal symptom relief produced by antihistamines improves the lung functions of many people with asthma.

TECHNICAL STUFF

Mast cells (among the cells that line your nose and respiratory tract) produce and release a chemical substance called *histamine*. You may only become aware of histamine when your immune system releases massive amounts of this chemical into your nasal tissue as a reaction to injury or in the presence of an allergen. After being released from the mast cells, histamine seeks out "receptor" sites located in the nasal lining tissues.

As we discuss in these sections, many antihistamine products are available, but they don't all work the same. Therefore, using the right antihistamine at the right dosage schedule will result in the best control of your allergy symptoms.

Using them for prevention

Many people tend to use antihistamines only as rescue medication. However, these products usually work much better and provide greater relief when they're taken preventively. Taking an antihistamine to relieve your symptoms is like closing the barn door after your horse has already bolted. You're not going to get that horse back in the barn (although by closing the door, you at least prevent any others from escaping).

TIP

Antihistamines usually work best when taken on a regular basis before allergen exposure occurs. For example:

>> If you're allergic to ragweed pollen, start using your medication at the beginning of August — before ragweed pollens are released in the middle of the month — and continue using the medication until after ragweed season is over. Even if you're exposed to significant amounts of allergen, you usually experience far fewer symptoms by using this type of preventive approach.

>> If you know that animal dander triggers your allergic rhinitis and you plan to visit someone who has pets, take your antihistamine two to five hours beforehand. Also, remember to continue with the antihistamine after you leave, until you have an opportunity to change your clothing, because dander is probably on your clothes.

Recognizing first-generation OTC antihistamines

The most common antihistamine medications are first-generation nonprescription products that are available in OTC form. Numerous nonprescription antihistamine products line drugstore and supermarket shelves. Most of these products, however, are just different brand names for a few of the same active ingredients, such as

>> **Brompheniramine maleate:** The active ingredient in Dimetapp

>> **Chlorpheniramine maleate:** The active ingredient in Chlor-Trimeton

>> **Clemastine fumarate:** The active ingredient in Dayhist

>> **Diphenhydramine hydrochloride:** The active ingredient in Benadryl

WARNING

Although first-generation OTC antihistamines can relieve allergic rhinitis symptoms such as sneezing, runny nose, and itchy nose, eyes, and throat, they also produce side effects that can significantly interfere with your daily life. These OTC antihistamines can cross from the bloodstream into your brain, where they affect histamine receptors in the central nervous system, resulting in drowsiness — the most serious and potentially dangerous side effect.

WARNING

Consider these factors when taking nonprescription antihistamines:

>> Many states in the United States consider people who take first-generation OTC antihistamines to be under the influence of drugs. The Federal Aviation Administration prohibits pilots from flying if they take OTC antihistamines within 24 hours of flight time. Similar restrictions on the use of first-generation OTC antihistamines apply to truck and bus drivers and operators in other transportation industries.

>> Operating heavy machinery or engaging in activities that require alertness, coordination, dexterity, or quick reflexes while taking first-generation OTC antihistamines is dangerous.

>> Avoid alcohol, sedatives, antidepressants, or other types of tranquilizers while taking first-generation OTC antihistamines.

>> First-generation OTC antihistamines can produce other side effects, including the following:

- Dizziness

- Dryness of mouth and sinus passages

- Gastrointestinal irritation or distress

- Nasal stuffiness

- Urine retention (which can aggravate existing prostate problems)

>> Recent studies show that children with allergic rhinitis who take diphen-hydramine hydrochloride (the active ingredient in Benadryl) for their symptoms score significantly lower on learning ability tests than children who receive equivalent doses of loratadine (the second-generation OTC antihistamine Claritin).

Identifying newer antihistamines

Due to significant advances in research since the development of first-generation antihistamines more than 60 years ago, several of the newer second-generation antihistamines have fewer side effects. Some of the benefits of these second-generation medications include

>> They don't cross the blood-brain barrier at recommended doses, which means that second-generation products such as loratadine (Alavert and

Claritin), and desloratadine (Clarinex) are considered nonsedating. However, fexofenadine (Allegra) is truly nonsedating and doesn't cross the blood-brain barrier at all. Alternatively, cetirizine (Zyrtec) and levocetirizine (Xyzal), are mildly sedating and may cause some sedative effects in certain individuals.

>> Side effects other than drowsiness, such as dry mouth, constipation, urine retention, or blurred vision, occur less frequently or are much less noticeable with second-generation antihistamines.

>> Although second-generation antihistamines, whether prescription or OTC (such as loratadine), can cost more than most first-generation nonprescription antihistamine products, the more recently developed products work longer and require only one or two doses per day to prevent or relieve allergic rhinitis symptoms.

>> For the most part, second-generation products work as rapidly as the first-generation drugs. For example, fexofenadine (Allegra), desloratadine (Clarinex), loratadine (Claritin), cetirizine (Zyrtec), and levocetirizine (Xyzal) usually start functioning within 1 to 3 hours.

>> Overall, patients who use second-generation antihistamines usually experience much less disruption or impairment in their daily lives.

Because of these factors, second-generation antihistamines (see Table 6-1) can greatly improve the treatment of allergic rhinitis. Allergic patients are far more likely to stick with second-generation antihistamines for the prescribed course, which often results in more effective prevention of allergic rhinitis symptoms.

TABLE 6-1   **Second-Generation Prescription (and OTC) Antihistamines**

Active Ingredient	Formulation	Brand Name	Total Usual Daily Dose for Children under 12 Years (See Formulation Details)	Total Usual Daily Adult Dose
Cetirizine	5 mg, 10 mg tablet (ages 12 years and older); 5 mg/5 ml syrup (2-5 years)	Zyrtec	Syrup, 2-5 years of age: ½ teaspoon (2.5 ml) daily; 6-11 years of age: 1-2 teaspoons (5-10 ml) daily	1 tablet once per day
Cetirizine (with 120 mg pseudoephedrine)	5 mg tablet (12 years and older)	Zyrtec-D	Not approved for children under 12 years of age	1 tablet twice per day
Desloratadine	5 mg tablet (12 years and older)	Clarinex	Not approved for children under 12 years of age	1 tablet once per day
Fexofenadine	30 mg/5 ml syrup	Children's Allegra	1 teaspoon (5 ml) every 12 hours (for ages 2-12 years)	2 teaspoons (10 ml) every 12 hours

Active Ingredient	Formulation	Brand Name	Total Usual Daily Dose for Children under 12 Years (See Formulation Details)	Total Usual Daily Adult Dose
Fexofenadine	30 mg tablet (6–11 years)	Allegra-Pediatric	1 tablet twice per day	2 tablets twice per day
Fexofenadine	60 mg capsule, 60 mg tablet (12 years and older)	Allegra	Not approved for children under 12 years of age	1 capsule twice per day 1 tablet twice per day
Fexofenadine	180 mg tablet (12 years and older)	Allegra-24 Hour	Not approved for children under 12 years of age	1 tablet once per day
Fexofenadine (with 120 mg pseudoephedrine)	60 mg tablet (12 years and older)	Allegra-D	Not approved for children under 12 years of age	1 tablet twice per day
Levocetirizine	5 mg tablet (12 years and older) Oral solution 2.5 mg/5ml	Xyzal	Oral solution (2–11 years of age) 2–5 years of age: ½ teaspoon (2.5 ml) at night 6–11 years of age: 1 teaspoon (5 ml) at night	1 tablet at bedtime or 1–2 teaspoons (5–10 ml) at bedtime
Loratadine	10 mg tablet (rapidly disintegrating) (6 years and older)	Alavert	1 tablet once per day (6 years and older)	1 tablet once per day
Loratadine	10 mg tablet (6 years and older)	Claritin	1 tablet once per day (6 years and older)	1 tablet once per day
Loratadine	10 mg tablet (rapidly disintegrating) (6 years and older)	Claritin RediTabs	1 tablet once per day (6 years and older)	1 tablet once per day
Loratadine	5 mg/5 ml syrup	Children's Claritin Syrup	2–6 years of age: 1 teaspoon (5 ml) daily over 6 years of age: 2 teaspoons (10 ml) daily	2 teaspoons (10 ml) daily
Loratadine (with 120 mg pseudoephedrine)	5 mg tablet (12 years and older)	Claritin-D 12 Hour	Not approved for children under 12 years of age	1 tablet twice per day
Loratadine (with 240 mg pseudoephedrine)	10 mg tablet (12 years and older)	Claritin-D 24 Hour	Not approved for children under 12 years of age	1 tablet once per day

mg = milligram; ml = milliliter

The names, formulations, and doses in the following table are evidence-based recommendations, which can change at any time. This table is designed to provide you with an overview of the second-generation antihistamines, but of course, you should discuss your individual needs with your physician.

Considering antihistamine nasal sprays

The names, formulations, and doses in the following list are evidence-based recommendations, which can change at any time. This list is designed to provide you with an overview of antihistamine nasal sprays, but of course, you should discuss your individual needs with your physician.

On the front lines of allergic rhinitis treatment, additions to the antihistamine arsenal in the United States are *azelastine hydrochloride* and *olopatadine hydrochloride*. Remember these basic facts about these nasal sprays:

>> Azelastine and olopatadine hydrochloride are highly effective for the treatment of seasonal allergic rhinitis symptoms such as sneezing, runny nose, nasal congestion, and itchy nose, eyes, and throat.

>> Studies show that, in contrast to most oral antihistamines, azelastine and olopatadine often help reduce nasal congestion (stuffy nose), which may make them particularly useful in dealing with the congestion that often accompanies allergic rhinitis due to late-phase reactions (delayed reaction, see Chapter 4).

>> You can use azelastine and olopatadine nasal sprays in combination treatment with nasal corticosteroid sprays in cases that require more prevention or relief. (See "Using nasal corticosteroids," later in this chapter, for more information on these sprays.)

>> The recommended dosage for azelastine and olopatadine is 2 sprays in each nostril twice a day for patients older than 12 and 1 spray in each nostril twice a day for children ages 6 to 11.

>> These sprays usually start to take effect within 3 hours.

>> The U.S. Food and Drug Administration (FDA) approved azelastine for the treatment of *vasomotor rhinitis* (nonallergic rhinitis; refer to the related sidebar in this chapter) for patients who are 12 or older. The recommended dosage is 2 sprays in each nostril twice a day.

>> Side effects of azelastine and olopatadine may include a bitter taste and drowsiness.

>> Olopatadine (Patanase) is a prescription intranasal antihistamine supplied in a white plastic bottle with a metered-dose manual spray pump. Patanase may cause sleepiness or drowsiness.

>> The FDA approved azelastine (Astepro) to be used without a prescription in patients who are 6 or older. For adults and children older than 12, the dose is 1 to 2 sprays in each nostril once or twice daily. For children ages 6 to 11, dosing is 1 spray in each nostril every 12 hours.

Decongesting Your Nose

People commonly use *decongestants* to relieve their stuffy noses. You can find two types of decongestants: oral decongestants in tablet, capsule, or liquid form, and nasal decongestants in the form of nasal sprays or nose drops. Unlike antihistamines, no second-generation decongestants have yet been developed. We discuss those two types in greater detail here.

Oral decongestants

Nonprescription oral decongestants are among the most widely used OTC products in the world, and you can find them in various tablet, capsule, or liquid forms. These medications work by shrinking blood vessels, thus reducing the amount of fluid that leaks into tissues lining the nose and decreasing nasal congestion. The most commonly used decongestants are *pseudoephedrine* and *phenylephrine.*

Pseudoephedrine is the active ingredient in OTC oral decongestants such as Sudafed, and in antihistamine-decongestant combinations such as Actifed and Dimetapp. This drug is the "D" (standing for decongestant) in the commonly used second-generation antihistamine products known as Allegra-D, Claritin-D, and Zyrtec-D.

WARNING

Be aware of the following information before using this type of decongestant:

>> Systemic decongestants are often combined with other drugs, such as antihistamines, *antipyretics* (fever reducers), *analgesics* (pain relievers), *antitussives* (cough suppressants), or *expectorants* (mucus loosener), to provide multi-symptom relief for headaches, fever, cough, sleeplessness, and other symptoms of the common cold, flu, allergic rhinitis, and other ailments.

>> Oral forms of systemic decongestants used consistently can cause side effects such as sleeplessness, nervous agitation, loss of appetite, dryness of mouth and sinuses, difficulty urinating, high blood pressure, and heart palpitations.

If you have a medical condition such as arrhythmia, coronary heart disease, hypertension, hyperthyroidism, glaucoma, diabetes, enlarged prostate, or urinary dysfunction, don't take any product containing a decongestant without first checking with your physician.

>> Because of the stimulant effect of oral decongestants, use caution when giving them to children. (Believe it or not, most parents aren't interested in unduly stimulating their kids.)

Nasal decongestants

Nonprescription decongestant nasal sprays and nose drops can provide quick and effective short-term relief of nasal congestion. However, you should use them only occasionally, and not for more than three to five days in a row, because long-term or consistent use can result in adverse effects such as *nasal rebound* (see the nearby sidebar).

WARNING

Never use decongestant nasal sprays and drops in children under the age of 6 without a physician's supervision. If you use them properly, OTC decongestants generally produce few side effects other than occasional sneezing and dry nasal passages. The most common OTC decongestant drugs and brand-name medications include

>> **Naphazoline,** found in Privine

>> **Oxymetazoline,** found in Afrin, Allerest, Dristan Long Lasting, and Sinex Long Lasting

>> **Phenylephrine,** found in Neo-Synephrine, Sinex, and Little Remedies Decongestant Nose Drops (0.125 percent formula for infants and children)

>> **Xylometazoline,** found in Otrivin

The dosage levels and usage frequency of these medications vary depending on each product's formulation and method of application. As always, carefully read all product instructions and warnings before using any medication.

The long-lasting products require no more than two doses a day to remain effective, but the short-acting products may work for only 1 to 4 hours. Therefore, you may need to apply short-acting products several times a day, as long as you don't exceed safe dosage levels and don't use the product continuously without checking first with your physician.

NASAL REBOUND

No, nasal rebound isn't a new basketball strategy. This condition, more formally known as *rhinitis medicamentosa,* results from prolonged overuse of OTC decongestant nasal sprays and drops. Overusing such medications can irritate and inflame the mucous membranes in your nose more than before you used the spray, leading to more serious nasal congestion.

Unfortunately, some people increase their use of the product as their congestion worsens, leading to a vicious cycle in which more use produces more congestion. When this happens, higher doses don't clear the congestion — they only make it worse. To break this vicious cycle, stop using your OTC decongestant. Your physician may also need to prescribe a short course of oral or nasal corticosteroids to clear your nasal congestion and allow you to tolerate the discontinuation of the OTC decongestant.

Remember, the warning on the label that directs you not to use nasal decongestant spray or drops longer than three to five days really means three to five days and no more. If your stuffy nose persists beyond that point, consider using an oral decongestant.

Two for the Nose: Combination Products

Antihistamines and decongestants can often be more effective in treating the full range of allergic rhinitis symptoms if you combine them in one preparation. You can find numerous oral OTC combination products in tablet, capsule, or liquid form on store shelves.

An antihistamine, such as chlorpheniramine or brompheniramine, is often combined with a decongestant, such as pseudoephedrine. These products are also frequently combined with other active ingredients — pain relievers, cough suppressants, and fever reducers, for example — to provide relief for a variety of ailments, such as cold and flu symptoms.

The onset of relief and dosage frequency vary with different products. Tablets and capsules generally come in two varieties:

>> **Rapid release:** These medications start working quickly but usually lose effectiveness within four hours.

>> **Sustained release:** As you may expect, these products work the opposite way: They act slower but last longer than rapid release medications — usually six to eight hours or longer.

Nondrowsy OTC formulas may contain pain relievers, fever reducers, cough suppressants, or other active ingredients for multisymptom relief but don't contain first-generation antihistamines, which cause drowsiness. Therefore, these formulas don't usually provide relief from the sneezing, runny nose, and itchy nose, eyes, and throat that are significant symptoms of allergic rhinitis.

WARNING

The decongestant in combination products can still cause sleeplessness, nervous agitation, loss of appetite, dryness of mouth and sinuses, high blood pressure, and heart palpitations, especially in older patients. Likewise, the antihistamine in combination products can still cause drowsiness. For example, the antihistamine diphenhydramine (Benadryl) is the active ingredient in many popular sleep aids, such as Nytol and Sominex.

In the next section, we discuss the different effects of antihistamines and decongestants, including the potential benefits and drawbacks of combining these medications, and why your physician will carefully consider the most appropriate option to treat your specific needs when prescribing a combined product.

Analyzing the upside and downside

Because of their sedative effects, OTC antihistamines are generally thought of as *downers*. Likewise, because decongestants act as stimulants, they're considered *uppers*. You may think that combining these two types of drugs in a single OTC product cancels out both the sedative and stimulant side effects. However, a person may experience both the upper and the downer effects at the same time — the worst of both worlds, in other words — resulting in an agitated, jittery form of drowsiness.

If a patient's condition warrants a combination product, their physician usually prescribes a nonsedating antihistamine formulated with a decongestant, such as Allegra-D, or possibly a less sedating antihistamine formulated with a decongestant, such as Zyrtec-D. The decongestant (pseudoephedrine) in these products usually doesn't produce as much of a stimulant effect as other decongestants, such as phenylpropanolamine, which the FDA removed from the market. As a result, the patient gets the benefits of both a nonsedating antihistamine and a less stimulating decongestant, minimizing the adverse downer or upper side effects.

TIP

Most OTC liquid forms are short-acting, which means they typically require up to four doses a day. However, you may prefer to use liquids, especially syrup forms that contain flavorings (and sometimes sweeteners), to treat children as well as adults who have trouble swallowing tablets and capsules. Another option is to use chewable formulations of these products.

One-size-fits-all may not suit your condition

Although combination antihistamine and decongestant products may work well when you need quick relief, the products are less suitable for long-term use because you can't adjust the dosage levels of the individual active ingredients. Each dose, whether in tablet, capsule, or liquid form, delivers the same amount of antihistamine and decongestant (as well as other active ingredients) to your system whether you need relief from one symptom or the full range of ailments.

WARNING

If you're considering switching combination products because the one you're using doesn't seem effective, check the active ingredients on other medications to make sure you don't buy the same antihistamine and decongestant combination under a different brand name.

Understanding the Advantages of Nasal Sprays

Targeting the exact location of a medical condition is preferable to treating the whole body with a systemic medication and hoping the affected area will somehow benefit from a wide spectrum approach. When treating allergic rhinitis, the advantage of using a nasal spray rather than an oral medication is that the spray directs the medication appropriately to the lining of the nasal passages.

This targeted treatment provides the greatest benefit of the medication in relieving nasal allergy symptoms, such as sneezing, itchy nose, runny nose, and nasal congestion, while still minimizing potential side effects. The bottom line is that using targeted medical therapy is safer and more effective to improve your nasal symptoms rather than medicating your entire body with the use of oral medications.

Here we discuss the role of nasal corticosteroids in managing allergic rhinitis symptoms. You discover how they work to suppress inflammation and clear nasal passages and the importance of using them daily for optimal results, We also explain how these medications are formulated to provide effective symptom relief and share tips for safe and convenient application.

Using nasal corticosteroids

The most effective medication currently available for controlling the four major symptoms of allergic rhinitis — sneezing, itching, runny nose, and nasal congestion — is *nasal corticosteroid spray*. Patients and the general public commonly refer to these corticosteroid products as *steroids* or *cortisone*. However, in this book, we use the proper term *corticosteroid* for these types of nasal sprays to avoid confusion.

The negative perception some people have of steroids is mostly due to attempts by some athletes to build up muscle mass by abusing *anabolic steroids*. In fact, the steroids used in corticosteroid nasal sprays are a completely different type of drug than anabolic steroids (which are actually male hormones).

REMEMBER

The spray is administered by an *aqueous* (non-aerosol) mechanical pump. The following information can help you and your physician decide whether nasal corticosteroids can work for you:

>> Nasal corticosteroid sprays suppress the inflammation of nasal passages, thereby clearing your nose for easier breathing.

>> Nasal corticosteroid sprays are most effective if you use them daily as preventive medications. For a guide to safe dosage levels, see Table 6-2.

>> Don't exceed the maximum recommended nasal spray dosage levels with these products to minimize any possibility of the medication causing systemic side effects associated with oral corticosteroids.

>> Nasal corticosteroid sprays provide gradual relief of allergic rhinitis symptoms. Initially, you may need to use the medication for several days before the spray suppresses your nasal inflammation. Full effectiveness may require two to three weeks of daily application.

>> Use nasal corticosteroids only if your nose is clear enough for the spray to penetrate. If your nose is seriously congested, you may need to use a nasal decongestant for the first three to five days just prior to administering the nasal corticosteroid spray.

>> To avoid injuring your *septum* (the bone that divides the nose into two nostrils), direct the spray away from your septum and slightly toward your ears. You may even want to spray the product once in the air to judge the force of the spray before using it in your nose.

>> Because of its gentler action on the nasal lining, using an aqueous formulation can minimize the typical adverse side effects of nasal corticosteroid sprays, such as nasal irritation, burning, drying, and nosebleeds.

SEE YOUR DOCTOR

The names, formulations, and doses in Table 6-2 are evidence-based recommendations, which can change at any time. Many of the branded nasal sprays are now available in generic form. For further information, check with your pharmacist or physician. This table isn't intended to provide medical advice. Of course, you should always discuss your individual needs with your physician.

TABLE 6-2 **Nasal Corticosteroid Sprays**

Active Ingredient	Formulation	Brand Name	Total Usual Daily Dose for Children under 12 Years (See Formulation Details)	Total Usual Daily Adult Dose
Budesonide	32 mcg per inhalation	Rhinocort Allergy Spray	1–2 sprays each nostril once per day (6–11 years)	1–2 sprays each nostril once per day
Fluticasone	50 mcg per inhalation	Flonase Allergy Relief Flonase Sensimist	1 spray each nostril once per day; may be increased to 2 sprays each nostril once per day (4–11 years)	2 sprays each nostril once per day or 1 spray each nostril twice per day; may be decreased to maintenance dose of 1 spray each nostril once per day
Fluticasone	93 mcg per inhalation	XHANCE	18 years of age and older	Prescription only Approved for treatment of nasal polyps 1–2 sprays each nostril twice per day
Mometasone	50 mcg per inhalation	Nasonex Allergy Nasal Spray	1 spray each nostril once per day; may be increased to 2 sprays each nostril once per day (3–11 years)	2 sprays each nostril once per day
Triamcinolone	55 mcg per inhalation	Nasacort 24-Hour Nasal Allergy Spray	2 sprays each nostril once per day (6–11 years)	2 sprays each nostril once per day

mcg = microgram

Trying combination nasal sprays

Studies have compared the combination of fluticasone and azelastine (Dymista) to its individual components and a *placebo* (an inactive substance) in patients 12 and older with at least a two-year history of seasonal allergic rhinitis. The studies showed that the combination of a nasal corticosteroid with a nasal antihistamine was superior to a nasal corticosteroid alone. The combination spray led to quicker symptom relief and better control than either medication alone.

Therefore, patients suffering from seasonal allergies may want to try a combination spray if a nasal corticosteroid alone isn't adequate. The two combinations available by prescription are the following:

>> **Azelastine and fluticasone (Dymista):** This combination nasal spray, also available as a generic product, works well to treat seasonal allergies for adults

and children 6 and older. The combination of azelastine, an antihistamine, and fluticasone, a corticosteroid that decreases swelling and inflammation in the nose, is usually prescribed when symptoms don't improve with intranasal steroid medications alone. The typical dose is 1 spray in each nostril twice daily.

>> **Olopatadine and mometasone (Ryaltis):** This combination nasal spray is prescribed to treat symptoms of allergic rhinitis. Olopatadine is an antihistamine, which prevents the effects of histamine, and mometasone is a corticosteroid, which has anti-inflammatory effects. The dose for adults and children over 12 is 2 sprays in each nostril twice per day.

WARNING

Although some evidence indicates that nasal corticosteroid sprays are highly effective and safe for children, some physicians are concerned about the possible effects the sprays may temporarily have on the growth rate of children who use them. If your child uses a nasal corticosteroid spray, make sure their physician knows about your concerns so they can accurately monitor your youngster's growth.

WARNING

CORTICOSTEROIDS TO AVOID

Although nasal corticosteroid sprays are highly effective and generally safe for both adults and children when administered under a physician's care, using other forms of steroids is less advisable and potentially unsafe. The following steroids may be harmful to you:

- **Oral corticosteroids:** We often using quick bursts of short-acting oral corticosteroids (such as prednisone or methylprednisolone) only in cases of severe nasal rebound or nasal polyps, where a decongestant nasal spray can't penetrate sufficiently to decongest your nose. In such cases, you may require a short course of oral corticosteroids prescribed by your physician to sufficiently clear your congestion so you can use a nasal corticosteroid spray.

- **Intranasal injections:** Cortisone shots into the nose aren't appropriate treatment for allergic rhinitis because of the potential for serious side effects, including vision complications and possibly even blindness.

Controlling Symptoms with Cromolyn Sodium

Cromolyn sodium, an anti-inflammatory OTC nasal spray, may be highly effective in controlling symptoms of allergic rhinitis when you use it properly. (You can find this medicine under the brand name NasalCrom.) Cromolyn sodium stabilizes mast cells, thereby preventing the release of histamine and other chemical mediators that can cause nasal inflammation.

TIP

To help determine whether cromolyn sodium nasal spray can work for you, check out these facts about its recommended use and effectiveness:

» Cromolyn sodium is most effective if you start using it two to four weeks before exposure to allergens. In cases of occupational allergic rhinitis or limited exposure to allergens, using the spray immediately prior to an isolated, single allergen exposure (before mowing the lawn or visiting a home with a pet) may provide some relief if your nasal passages aren't already congested.

» If allergic rhinitis symptoms are already present, you may need a short course of a combination antihistamine-decongestant for the first few days you use cromolyn sodium.

» You can purchase cromolyn sodium in a metered spray form. The recommended dosage for adults and children older than 6 is 1 spray in each nostril, 3 to 6 times per day, at regular intervals. Administer cromolyn sodium to children between 2 and 6 years of age only under the supervision of a physician.

TREATING HAY FEVER SYMPTOMS IN PREGNANT WOMEN

Physicians often recommend nasal saline irrigation as a first line treatment option for the management of allergic rhinitis symptoms in pregnant women. Oral antihistamines (such as cetirizine) are also considered to be a safe and effective option.

Recent guidelines recommend that pregnant women should avoid oral decongestants during the first trimester of pregnancy, but your physician may prescribe nasal decongestant sprays (Afrin, Neo-Synephrine) and topic nasal corticosteroids (Flonase) for short-term relief from the second trimester onward.

Always consult your physician before starting any new medication while pregnant (check out Dr. Berger's *Asthma For Dummies* [John Wiley & Sons, Inc.] for more information on this topic).

Reducing Mucus with Anticholinergic Sprays

Ipratropium bromide is the active ingredient in the *anticholinergic products* (drying agents) that sell under the brand name Atrovent Nasal Spray. Anticholinergics counter cholinergic activity by blocking *acetylcholine* — a neurotransmitter that stimulates mucus production — from attaching to chemical receptors in the nose. Therefore, these sprays reduce the amount of mucus in your nose.

Some basic facts about anticholinergic sprays include

>> Ipratropium bromide effectively reduces runny nose, as seen in conditions such as *vasomotor* (nonallergic rhinitis; see the nearby sidebar) or the common cold.

>> Ipratropium bromide has little effect on other allergic rhinitis symptoms, such as stuffy nose, sneezing, or itchy nose.

>> Your physician can prescribe Atrovent Nasal Spray in two strengths: 0.03 percent for relief of runny nose associated with allergic and nonallergic rhinitis in adults and children older than 6, and 0.06 percent for relief of runny nose associated with the common cold in adults and children older than 12.

>> The typical dose is 2 sprays per nostril 2 or 3 times per day (0.03 percent) or 3 or 4 times per day (0.06 percent) at regular intervals.

PREVENTING SKIER'S NOSE

Ever notice how often skiers blow their noses? You may have seen several boxes of tissues at the bottom of the ski lifts at your favorite resort. The tissues are there because of what people call *skier's nose,* which is triggered by cold air and is symptomatic of *vasomotor rhinitis* (inflammation of the nasal tissues that is triggered by environmental factors such as strong odors, cold air, alcohol ingestion, and spicy foods).

Atrovent Nasal Spray works well to prevent skier's nose as well as jogger's nose, if you use it before being exposed to cold air, and also for treatment after symptoms appear. However, physicians also use anticholinergic eye drops similar to ipratropium bromide (the active ingredient in Atrovent) to dilate patients' eyes, so make sure you keep the spray away from your eyes or you won't see that mogul coming right at you.

Treating Rhinitis with Leukotriene Modifiers

Leukotrienes play a significant role in asthma attacks. These chemicals, found in the mast cells that line the airways of the lungs and nose, enhance mucus production, constrict the bronchial passages, and promote further inflammation of the respiratory lining by attracting additional inflammatory cells into the airways.

Leukotriene modifiers, such as *montelukast* (Singulair), approved for the treatment of asthma, are drugs that block leukotriene activity at the receptor site, thus decreasing the amount of mucus generated by exposure to allergens.

WARNING

Leukotriene modifiers may be used to treat patients whose allergic rhinitis symptoms don't respond solely to antihistamines. However, the FDA requires a *black box warning* (used for medications that carry serious safety risks) for montelukast (Singulair) because of the risk of neuropsychiatric events (mental side effects) associated with this drug. The warning advises healthcare providers to avoid prescribing montelukast for patients with mild allergic rhinitis.

Keeping an Eye Out for Allergic Conjunctivitis

Allergic conjunctivitis often coexists with allergic rhinitis. In fact, most of the same allergens involved in allergic rhinitis can trigger allergic conjunctivitis. Characteristic symptoms of this ailment include redness of the eyes and the underside of the eyelids, and swollen, itchy, and watery eyes.

REMEMBER

Because the mechanisms of allergic rhinitis and allergic conjunctivitis are similar, conjunctivitis is often treated with some of the same types of drugs used to control rhinitis in solutions specifically formulated for safe use in the eye. Treatment can include

>> **Prescription antihistamines:** Two newer second-generation prescription antihistamines, *levocabastine* (Livostin) and *emedastine* (Emadine), appear to be more effective than OTC antihistamines for the treatment of allergic conjunctivitis. Normal recommended dosage for both products is 1 drop per eye up to 4 times a day for up to 2 weeks.

>> **OTC decongestants:** Products include Clear Eyes, Clear Eyes ACR, Visine A.C., Visine L.R., Visine Moisturizing, and Visine Original.

>> **Combinations of OTC antihistamines and decongestants:** Products include Naphcon-A, Vasocon-A, Ocuhist, Prefrin, and VasoClear.

>> **Mast cell stabilizers:** This group of medications, available by prescription, inhibits mast cells from releasing chemical mediators of inflammation, potentially preventing allergic symptoms from developing. These types of eye-drop products include

- **Cromolyn sodium (Crolom, Opticrom):** Cromolyn sodium works best if you use it preventively, prior to allergen exposure, but you also can administer it on a regular basis, four times a day. For infrequent allergen exposure (when visiting someone with pets, for example), use cromolyn sodium immediately before you expect to be exposed to the allergen. This product has also demonstrated some effectiveness in treating forms of *vernal conjunctivitis* (a chronic eye condition that can cause severe burning and intense itching and marked sensitivity to bright light).

- **Nedocromil sodium (Alocril):** This medication, available in a metered-dose inhaler formulation for the treatment of asthma (Tilade), is also approved in the United States as an *ophthalmic* (eye) solution. Physicians can prescribe it for itching eyes associated with allergic conjunctivitis in adults and children as young as 3. This product provides effective relief of both the early and late-phase allergic response (delayed reaction). The normal dosage for Alocril is 1 or 2 drops in each eye twice per day.

- **Lodoxamide (Alomide):** This drug isn't approved for use specifically for allergic conjunctivitis, but it has shown some effectiveness in clinical trials as a treatment for vernal conjunctivitis. Normal dosage is 1 or 2 drops per eye, 4 times per day, for up to 3 months.

>> **Nonsteroidal anti-inflammatory drugs (NSAIDs):** Ketorolac (Acular) is a type of NSAID that can relieve the itching of seasonal allergic conjunctivitis. Normal dosage is 1 drop per eye, 4 times per day.

>> **Combination antihistamine and mast cell stabilizer:** The most recent additions to allergic conjunctivitis eye products are olopatadine (Patanol, Pataday OTC) and ketotifen (Zaditor OTC), which are available OTC, and azelastine (Optivar Rx) and epinastine (Elestat Rx), which are available by prescription in the United States. The normal recommended dosage for Patanol is one drop in each affected eye twice per day, at an interval of six to eight hours. For Zaditor, the recommended dosage is 1 drop in each eye twice daily, every 8 to 12 hours. The recommended dosage for Optivar and also for Elestat is 1 drop in each eye twice a day.

Physicians prescribe corticosteroid eye drops for severe cases of allergic conjunctivitis that are unresponsive to the medications we describe in the preceding bullet points. However, you should monitor your use of corticosteroid eye drops closely because using these products improperly can lead to very serious adverse side effects. Don't ever use corticosteroid eye drops if you suspect you have a viral infection of the eyes, such as herpes, because using these products may prolong the course of and increase the severity of the viral infection. In addition, prolonged use of corticosteroid eye drops may result in glaucoma, vision complications, and cataract formation. Consider consulting a qualified *ophthalmologist* (eye doctor) before routinely using corticosteroid eye products.

Patients with allergic conjunctivitis should use eye drops during peak pollination seasons in addition to their other prescribed medication for allergic rhinitis to minimize eye discomfort. Try not to rub your eyes. Even though they may itch, rubbing them usually only makes matters worse. Instead, gently rinsing your eyes with clean water or a soothing OTC sterile irrigating solution can often wash away pollen and help relieve your symptoms.

If you experience severe allergic conjunctivitis, your physician may prescribe an oral antihistamine, eye drops, or a combination of two different eye-drop products for maximum relief of your symptoms.

IN THIS CHAPTER

» Identifying your nasal symptoms and common causes

» Determining appropriate solutions to treat your nasal symptoms

» Evaluating and managing sinus infections

» Diagnosing ear infections and managing them effectively

» Becoming aware of complications of untreated or poorly managed allergies

Chapter **7**

Assessing Common Nasal Allergy Complications

I f you suffer from asthma, you may also suffer from seasonal allergies such as *allergic rhinitis* (hay fever). The multiple allergens that commonly trigger allergic rhinitis often aggravate or worsen the respiratory symptoms associated with asthma.

Extensive studies over the last 30 years have shown that patients with allergic asthma usually are more successful in managing their respiratory condition if they take effective measures to control their allergic rhinitis symptoms. Ineffective treatment of allergic rhinitis can lead to serious complications of allergic rhinitis, such as *sinusitis* (an inflammation of the sinuses) and *otitis media* (an inflammation of the middle ear).

Other conditions, such as *tonsillitis* (an inflammation of the tonsils), adenoid disease, and chronic cough, can be worsened by *postnasal drip* (nasal discharge that trickles down the back of your throat). This characteristic symptom of allergic rhinitis, which usually increases in severity when the ailment is poorly managed, can result in the spread of bacteria-laden mucus that irritates or infects the throat's lining.

In this chapter we discuss the common causes of nasal allergy complications, and treatment options for these conditions. We also discuss how you can make smart choices to effectively manage and minimize the impact of your allergic rhinitis symptoms to avoid additional complications of the ear, nose, and throat.

Describing Sinusitis

If you've ever had cold or nasal symptoms that didn't seem to go away, you may have been suffering from a form of *sinusitis*. This usually painful condition develops as a result of swollen nasal and sinus passages frequently caused by allergic rhinitis. Many asthma patients often confuse sinusitis symptoms with the symptoms of a cold, flu, or allergy.

Sinusitis is one of the most common health problems in the United States. Current estimates indicate that more than 30 million Americans are diagnosed with sinusitis each year. Because of the congestion and discomfort sinusitis causes, it's one of the most common reasons for doctor visits in the United States.

SEE YOUR DOCTOR

Consult a physician as soon as you suspect you may have sinusitis. Complications, such as aggravation of asthma, recurrent bronchitis, otitis media, and nasal polyps, can occur if you manage your sinusitis poorly. Chronic sinus infections can result in swollen *adenoids* (glands located in the upper airway just behind the nasal cavity) that may require surgery to remove. On a more positive note, studies show that asthma patients who effectively manage their sinusitis can significantly improve their respiratory symptoms.

In the following sections, we delve deeper into the causes of sinusitis and describe how your sinuses help defend you from infections. We also discuss how physicians classify and diagnose different cases of sinusitis, and we examine ways of managing the condition.

Recognizing common causes

In a significant number of sinusitis cases, allergic rhinitis precedes the start of a sinus infection. Research shows that more than half of all children in the United States who receive treatment for sinusitis also have allergic rhinitis.

TECHNICAL STUFF

Vasomotor rhinitis, a nonallergic form of rhinitis that results from sudden temperature changes or exposure to tobacco smoke, pollutants, and other irritants, can also contribute to sinusitis. Swimmers, divers, fliers (passengers as well as flight crews), and other people with this form of rhinitis who frequently experience pressure and weather changes may be particularly prone to developing sinusitis if they don't effectively manage their rhinitis symptoms.

Other factors (you may have one or more of these) that can increase your chances of developing sinusitis include

>> **Upper respiratory viral infections:** Viruses, such as those associated with the common cold, are the most frequent cause of sinusitis.

>> **Bacterial infections:** The same family of germs that can cause acute otitis media (*Streptococcus pneumoniae, Haemophilus influenzae, Moraxella catarrhalis*) can cause acute bacterial sinusitis. Unlike viral infections, this type of sinusitis responds to antibiotic therapy.

>> **Fungal infections:** This type of sinusitis infection can develop in otherwise healthy patients who have been on long-term antibiotic treatment or have been taking oral corticosteroids on a chronic basis. *Aspergillus* is the most common fungus that causes these types of cases and is also frequently implicated in cases of *allergic fungal sinusitis.* Characteristic signs and symptoms of this recurring fungal infection, which can often affect individuals with allergic rhinitis or asthma, are sinus infections and *nasal polyps* (growths in the nose).

>> **Nasal rebound:** Overuse of over-the-counter (OTC) topical nasal decongestants can predispose you to sinusitis. (See Chapter 6 for more information.)

>> **Anatomical obstructions:** Nasal polyps, other growths, enlarged adenoids (particularly in children), and a deviated *nasal septum* (the great divide between the nostrils) can increase your chances of developing sinusitis.

>> **Other diseases:** Patients with cystic fibrosis, in which abnormally thick mucus is produced and the function of the *cilia* (tiny hairlike projections of certain types of cells that sweep debris-laden mucus through the airways) is impaired, frequently suffer from sinus infections. In addition, HIV/AIDS and other immune-deficiency diseases often weaken the body's defenses to the point where bacteria and viruses can cause many types of infections, including sinusitis. Patients with compromised immune systems may be particularly

vulnerable to various forms of fungal sinus infections. There are some rare conditions, mainly in adults, where sinusitis can occur first and the infection is a result of the original sinus inflammation.

Exploring sinus science

Allergists refer to the sinuses that surround your nose — called *paranasal sinuses* — when they discuss sinusitis. *Para* is Greek for around or near; *nasal*, of course, refers to the nose; and *sinus* is Latin for a hollow place. Your sinuses are hollow cavities in the bones that surround your nasal cavity (see Figure 7-1) — hence *sinusitis*, which means inflammation (*itis*) of the sinuses.

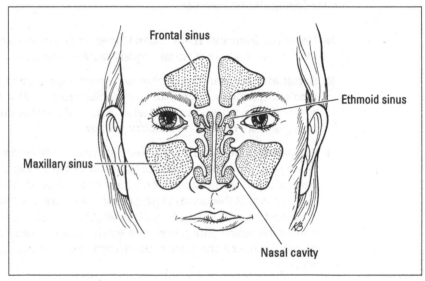

FIGURE 7-1:
Your sinuses are actually hollow cavities that surround your nasal cavity.

The three types of paranasal sinuses come in pairs (one on each side of the nose) and are named for the bones that house them. They include

>> **Maxillary sinuses:** The largest of the sinuses, these sinuses are located in your cheekbones.

>> **Frontal sinuses:** These sinuses reside in your forehead above your eyes.

>> **Ethmoid sinuses:** These sinuses are directly behind your eyes and nose.

The other sinus affected by sinusitis is the *sphenoid* sinus, located behind your nose near the base of your brain and may connect to the nose via the ethmoid sinuses.

TECHNICAL STUFF

Sinus infections usually affect the maxillary, frontal, and ethmoid sinuses. The most common complication affects the orbit around the eye, causing *cellulitis* (a potentially serious bacterial infection of the skin and the tissue beneath your skin) and possibly forming an *abscess* (a localized collection of pus surrounded by inflamed tissue). Patients with this type of infection may look as though they've taken a hard punch to the eye. Because the sphenoid sinus is near the brain, an infection in this area, although rare, is usually associated with infections in all the other sinuses (*pansinusitis*) and can have very serious consequences if infected fluids spread to the central nervous system. Untreated sinusitis has the potential to lead to life-threatening conditions, such as *meningitis* (an infection of the membranes that envelop the brain and spinal cord) and brain abscesses.

Understanding the purpose of sinuses

Your maxillary sinuses are present at birth, along with immature ethmoid sinuses, which begin to fully develop when you're between 3 and 7 years old. Therefore, contrary to previous medical opinion, children under 5 can experience sinus infections that require appropriate therapy. If your young child has allergic rhinitis, effectively treating their condition is vital in reducing their risk of developing sinusitis.

REMEMBER

Sinuses are a vital part of your body's defense against the airborne bacteria, viruses, irritants, and allergens you constantly inhale. Under normal circumstances, the mucus in your sinuses traps most of these intruders. Cilia sweep the particle-laden mucus through connecting *ostia* (sinus drainage openings) into your nasal passages, which drain it into your throat. From your throat, the mucus moves into your stomach, where your digestive system can neutralize and eventually eliminate the offending substances.

In addition to helping clear your upper respiratory tract of particle-laden mucus, your sinuses serve other important roles. For example, your sinuses act as

>> Air pockets that lighten your skull — otherwise, your head would be too heavy for your neck. Calling someone an airhead is actually an anatomically correct statement.

>> Resonance chambers that provide space for your voice to *resonate* (produce a full sound).

>> Climate adjusters, warming and humidifying the air you inhale.

>> Facial insulators, which also warm the base of your brain, located directly behind your nose.

>> Shock absorbers, protecting the inside of your skull from injury.

Allergic rhinitis irritates the nasal and sinus linings, causing them to swell, which narrows the sinus drainage openings into the nasal cavity. At the same time, your immune system's response to allergic rhinitis increases mucus production. This combination of increased mucus flow and a swollen sinus lining overwhelms the cilia's ability to sweep out the mucus, which then becomes infected.

Think of a swiftly flowing stream. If the stream dams up, the water usually stagnates and turns into a breeding ground for all sorts of organisms. The same process applies to your sinuses, which is why it's crucial to prevent them from turning into swamps.

Managing sinusitis

Although no universal definition exists for the various presentations of sinusitis, most physicians base their sinusitis classifications on the duration and types of symptoms involved. Therefore, physicians often use the following terms to classify cases of sinusitis:

>> **Acute sinusitis:** Symptoms of acute sinusitis persist for up to three or four weeks, although some physicians may diagnose symptoms that continue for up to eight weeks as acute. Typical symptoms of acute sinusitis include

- Upper respiratory infection.

- Runny nose with infected mucus that often appears as cloudy, thick, yellowish, or greenish nasal discharge.

- Cloudy, yellowish, or greenish postnasal drip (often of such a quantity that you may need to swallow frequently).

- Facial pain or pressure around cheeks, eyes, and lower nose (mainly in adults, less commonly in children), especially while bending over or moving vigorously (for example, during exercise).

- Nasal congestion, headache, fever, and cough.

- A reduction or loss of the sense of smell, pain in the upper teeth or upper jawbone, and *halitosis* (bad breath).

- In some children, nausea and vomiting due to gagging on infected mucus. Some children have a persistent *nocturnal* (nighttime) cough and halitosis.

>> **Chronic sinusitis:** When your condition lasts longer than four weeks, physicians usually consider you a chronic sufferer. In many cases, chronic sinusitis can last for months with combinations of the same symptoms as acute sinusitis, although you may not have a fever. For this reason, many people with chronic sinusitis think they suffer from frequent or constant colds.

>> **Recurrent sinusitis:** Physicians usually define recurrent sinusitis as three or more episodes of acute sinusitis per year. The recurring episodes may have different causes. If you have recurrent sinusitis, your physician may refer you to an allergist to determine whether allergies are the underlying cause of your condition. Recurrent sinusitis may be due to an underlying primary immuno-deficiency disorder. The immunodeficiency diseases most commonly associated with recurrent and chronic sinusitis are antibody deficient states also known as *hypogammaglobulinemia.*

Diagnosing sinusitis

SEE YOUR DOCTOR

Often, your physician can diagnose sinusitis based on your symptoms and medical history. They may ask questions like the following:

>> When did you first notice the symptoms?

>> What hurts? Where do you feel the pain?

>> Does your family have a history of allergies and sinus problems?

>> What have you done to treat your symptoms? What types of medications have you taken, and what has been their effect?

Your physician also conducts a physical exam of your nose and sinuses to confirm the diagnosis. This exam may include

>> Taking your temperature to check for fever and listening to your chest to see whether the infection has spread to your lungs.

>> Lightly tapping your forehead and cheekbones to check for sensitivity in your frontal and maxillary sinuses.

>> Looking for infected mucus in your nose and the back of your throat. This exam may require insertion of a flexible fiber-optic device, known as an *endoscope,* or a fiber-optic *rhinopharyngoscope,* so they can clearly view potentially infected areas.

Your doctor may use sophisticated imaging techniques to confirm the diagnosis of sinusitis. *Computed tomography* (CT) is currently the gold standard and, in many cases, is replacing the use of less accurate sinus X-rays. A CT scan, also known as a *computed axial tomography (CAT) scan*, is a diagnostic test that combines X-rays with state-of-the-art computer technology. This test uses a series of X-ray beams from many different angles to create cross-sectional images of your body — in this case, of your head and sinuses. With computer assistance, these images are assembled into a three-dimensional picture that can display organs, bones, and tissues in great detail.

Determining the best course of treatment

To effectively treat your sinusitis, you need to effectively manage your allergic rhinitis. In many cases, appropriately treating your allergic rhinitis also improves your sinusitis. As we explain in Chapter 5, avoidance and allergy-proofing are crucial tools you can use to effectively treat your allergies. Chapter 6 provides an in-depth explanation of allergy medications that you may find appropriate for your condition.

In addition to addressing your allergic rhinitis, physicians can prescribe a variety of treatments for sinusitis, ranging from medication to irrigation to surgery.

Antibiotics

Antibiotics are the most common medications that doctors prescribe to clear up the bacterial (not viral) infection in your sinuses. When taking antibiotics, keep the following in mind:

>> Because the blood flow to your sinuses is poor, you may need to take your prescribed antibiotics for a while before you notice a beneficial effect. However, most cases of acute sinusitis respond to antibiotic treatment within two weeks.

>> In cases of chronic sinusitis, don't be surprised if your physician prescribes a six- to eight-week course of antibiotic therapy combined with intranasal steroids (see Chapter 6) to eliminate your bacterial infection.

>> In some cases of acute or chronic sinusitis, you may notice a sudden improvement in your symptoms soon after you start a course of antibiotics, and you may consider stopping the medication at that point. However, it's extremely important that you take the complete course of antibiotics to ensure that all the bacteria have been completely eliminated.

Other medications

SEE YOUR DOCTOR

In addition to prescribing antibiotics to clear up the bacterial infection in your sinuses, your physician may prescribe medications to treat symptoms of allergic rhinitis, which we describe extensively in Chapter 6. In some cases your physician may prescribe mupirocin nasal ointment, an antibiotic that treats and prevents bacterial infections in the nose. It works by killing or stopping the growth of bacteria such as staphylococcus aureus which may be found in the nasal cavity of patients who are carriers of these bacteria.

Irrigation

SEE YOUR DOCTOR

Your physician may advise you to irrigate your nasal passages, a process known as *nasal lavage,* using a nasal douche cup, nasal spray bottle, nasal bulb syringe, neti pot, Waterpik with nasal attachment, or some other type of nasal wash device to rinse your nostrils with warm saline solution. You can use these devices at home to relieve pressure and congestion in your nasal passages. Ask your physician for specific instructions on how to use nasal wash devices.

Getting steamed

Your physician may also recommend a simple home remedy to help clear your sinuses and relieve discomfort. This remedy consists of inhaling steam to liquefy and soften crusty mucus while moisturizing your inflamed passages.

TIP

Use the following method for inhaling steam:

1. Boil water in a kettle on the stove.

2. Carefully pour the boiling water into a pan or basin on a low table.

3. Sit at the table and drape a towel over your head, leaning over the pan or basin to form a kind of human tent with your head as the pole.

4. Hold your face a few inches above the steaming water and breathe the steam through your nose for approximately ten minutes.

Two steam treatments a day may provide relief. However, you still need to deal with the underlying cause of the sinus infection, so we don't advise relying on this home remedy as the only therapy for your infectious sinusitis.

REMEMBER

Also consider obtaining a steam inhaler, such as the MyPurMist Handheld Vaporizer and Humidifier, which converts water to vapor without the risk of being scalded by boiling water. This portable handheld steam inhaler produces a fine instant mist, which is temperature-controlled and provides relief from nasal and sinus symptoms.

Sinus surgery

If other treatment methods don't provide effective relief, you may need surgery, especially if physical obstructions, such as a deviated septum or nasal polyps, contribute to your condition. However, if allergic rhinitis is the underlying cause of your sinusitis, surgery alone won't resolve your sinus problems. You must continue managing your allergic rhinitis to avoid further complications. By the same token, treating your allergies alone won't reverse the damage that sinusitis may have already caused.

If your physician thinks surgery is advisable, they'll refer you to an ear, nose, and throat specialist, or ENT, otherwise known as an *otolaryngologist* (remember that word the next time you do a crossword puzzle). Before you consider surgery, make sure your physician thoroughly reviews your medical history and evaluates your clinical condition.

TIP

Never hesitate to ask your surgeon for further information about your planned surgical procedure, such as how long the procedure takes, where and when it will be performed, what the possible complications are, and how soon you can get back to work or school.

The good news about sinus surgery is that the two most common procedures are minimally invasive. An ENT can perform them on an outpatient basis with local anesthesia, although they may use general anesthesia in certain cases. The two procedures most often used are

>> **Antral puncture and irrigation:** This procedure opens your sinuses so they can drain and irrigate properly, but it's used less often since the advent of fiber-optic surgery.

>> **Functional endoscopic sinus surgery:** This procedure is more complex than antral puncture and irrigation. Functional endoscopic sinus surgery often involves enlarging the ethmoid and maxillary sinus openings into the nasal cavity and removing and cleaning the infected sinus membranes, resulting in improved drainage. This procedure reestablishes the ventilation of your ethmoid, maxillary, and frontal sinuses. Otolaryngologists perform this type of surgery with high-tech computer-assisted instruments and navigation devices to ensure pinpoint accuracy.

Taking preventive measures

TIP

If you have allergic rhinitis, consider the following preventive measures to keep your sinuses clear if you come down with an upper respiratory infection (such as the common cold) or experience an allergy attack:

>> **Take the appropriate medications.** See Chapter 6 for a complete listing.

>> **Drink plenty of water.** Water keeps your mucus thin and fluid so your sinuses can drain more easily.

>> **Be nice to your nose.** Blow it gently, preferably one nostril at a time.

>> **Avoid flying.** If you have to travel by air while you have a cold or an allergy attack, use a nasal decongestant spray prior to takeoff. The spray prevents the sudden pressure changes from blocking your sinuses and ears.

>> **Avoid swimming.** You probably won't feel like going to the beach or the pool if you have a cold or allergy attack, and your sinuses definitely won't enjoy the pressure changes that swimming and diving involve. (Scuba diving wouldn't be a good idea either.)

Overcoming Otitis Media

Otitis media is an inflammation of the middle ear, as well as a condition in which fluid accumulates in your ear. This condition is different from *otitis externa,* which affects the external auditory canal and is commonly known as *swimmer's ear.* Based on the definitions of sinusitis and rhinitis we provide in this chapter, you can probably already guess what *otitis* means: an inflammation (*itis*) of the ear (*otikos* in Greek). *Media* means middle, by the way. Infectious organisms, such as bacteria and viruses, often affect the middle ear. Otitis media can develop as a result of allergic rhinitis and from complications of sinusitis.

Middle ear infections and fluid in the ear are especially common in young children and infants. In fact, otitis media is the most common reason for pediatric visits in the United States, with physicians treating at least 10 million children annually for ear infections. Otitis media can have serious consequences for youngsters, in particular by adversely affecting their development and learning ability due to potential hearing loss.

The most common forms of otitis media are

>> **Acute otitis media (AOM):** This condition involves inflammation and infection of the middle ear and Eustachian tube (see "Getting an earful," later in the chapter, for more on the Eustachian tube). The peak incidence of AOM is between 6 months and 1 year of age, decreasing with age and with fewer episodes after age 7.

>> **Otitis media with effusion (OME):** Physicians also refer to this condition as *serous otitis media* — fluid in the middle ear. OME, which occurs commonly in children from age 2 to 7, can lead to hearing loss if not treated properly.

As in most medical conditions treating symptoms won't ensure consistent improvement. Therefore, in addition to making the correct diagnosis your physician, working with you, should do their best to identify the cause of your symptoms to achieve the best result possible.

Revealing common causes

In a significant number of cases, allergic rhinitis precedes an ear infection. A long-term study of 2,000 children found that 50 percent of the patients with chronic and recurrent ear infections who were 3 or older had allergic rhinitis.

Other conditions that can increase your chances of developing ear infections include

>> Sinusitis. The same factors that can lead to sinus infections, such as exposure to allergens, tobacco smoke, pollutants, and other irritants, can contribute to ear infections.

>> Enlarged adenoids.

>> Unrepaired cleft palate.

>> Nasal polyps.

>> Pacifier use by babies.

>> Defective or immature immune system.

>> Benign or malignant tumors.

>> Teething. Some physicians believe that teething in young children can contribute to ear infections, but no one has established a direct connection.

TIP

Many of the conditions in the previous list affect infants and young children. Always ask your physician to check for infection and fluid in the middle ear anytime your child is ill.

Getting an earful

The visible part of your ear — that funny-looking protrusion on the side of your head — is only the tip of the iceberg. Most of your ear's functions take place inside your skull in chambers, tubes, and passages that register and conduct sound and also provide your sense of balance. The following describes parts of the ear (see Figure 7-2):

>> **Outer ear:** Also known as the *pinna,* this structure is what many people think of as the ear. The primary function of this skin-covered flap of elastic cartilage is to funnel sound into the middle ear and keep your eyeglasses on the side of your head.

>> **Middle ear:** This air-filled chamber is bordered by the *tympanic membrane* (commonly known as the *eardrum*) and small bones that enable your eardrum to function. Through its connection (the *Eustachian tube*) to the *nasopharynx* (back of the nose), your middle ear also equalizes the air pressure on both sides of your eardrum.

>> **Inner ear:** Your inner ear contains sensory receptors that provide your hearing and balance. The hearing receptors are enclosed in the *cochlea,* a fluid-filled chamber, while the balance receptors are in the semicircular canals.

>> **Eustachian tube (ET):** The ET is an extension of the middle ear that connects to the nasopharynx. The ET, which is often the origin of ear infections, serves three important functions:

- The ET provides ventilation for your middle ear.

- The ET helps equalize air pressure inside your ear, buffering your eardrum from the force of external air, and helps disperse the energy of sound waves from your inner ear into your throat.

- Because your ET is closed most of the time, it serves as an important barrier to viruses, bacteria, irritants, and allergens that enter your middle ear. Similar to their function in your sinuses, cilia in the middle ear sweep debris-laden mucus from your middle ear through the ET into the back of your nasal cavity. The cilia prepare the mucus for drainage into your throat and eventually into your stomach.

  The ET briefly opens to allow the cilia to sweep mucus away when you swallow, yawn, sniff, or strain. In many children, however, the ET doesn't fully develop until age 6, causing it to ineffectively ventilate, clear, or protect the middle ear. Therefore, large numbers of young children get middle ear infections.

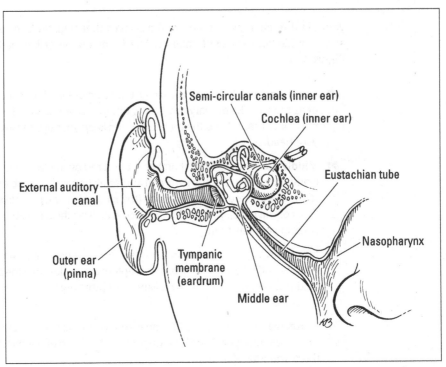

FIGURE 7-2:
See how the less
visible part of
your ear is
constructed.

© John Wiley & Sons, Inc.

Exploring acute otitis media

Many people suffer from *acute otitis media*, or AOM — an inflammation and infection of the middle ear and Eustachian tube — in early childhood. The main symptoms include

>> Earache — sometimes with intense, stabbing pains — and fever. Occasionally, vomiting and diarrhea accompany this symptom.

>> Possible hearing loss and occasional dizziness and ringing in the affected ear.

>> With infants, high fever, irritability, and a tendency to pull on the affected ear.

>> In some cases, discharge of infected fluid from the middle ear (if your eardrum has been perforated).

WARNING

An AOM infection generally develops as a result of an allergic, bacterial, or viral ailment that inflames your nose, sinuses, middle ear, and ET. Your ET may swell shut, trapping infected fluid, which then presses on your eardrum, causing the pain you associate with an earache. If you don't resolve this situation, infected fluids can eventually reach the membranes that cover your brain, leading to meningitis and even death.

Because sinusitis and otitis media often coexist, physicians usually treat these conditions with the same medications. Treatment of AOM often includes a course of antibiotics (available by prescription only) to rid your middle ear of infection. The antibiotic drugs that physicians commonly prescribe include

>> Amoxicillin (Amoxil) or amoxicillin/potassium clavulanate (Augmentin)

>> Clarithromycin (Biaxin) or azithromycin (Zithromax)

>> Trimethoprim-sulfamethoxazole (Bactrim or Septra)

>> A third-generation cephalosporin antibiotic, such as cefuroxime (Ceftin), cefpodoxime (Vantin), cefprozil (Cefzil), or cefixime (Suprax)

WARNING

If you're allergic to penicillin, make sure your doctor knows. Some people who have penicillin allergies may also have adverse reactions to cephalosporin medications.

Examining otitis media with effusion

When you have *otitis media with effusion,* or OME (also known as *serous otitis media*), your middle ear traps infected or sterile fluid. The most common symptoms of OME are

>> Plugged-up ears (similar to the discomfort you may experience when descending in an airplane)

>> Some hearing loss

TIP

Children with OME may not show obvious symptoms. However, if your child acts inattentive (other than the obvious times when children don't seem to hear you asking them to clean their room), doesn't seem to hear well (for example, they always want the television volume turned up loud), or talks loudly, make sure your physician examines their ears. Undetected or poorly treated OME can result in hearing loss, poor language development, learning disorders, and eventual behavioral problems.

OME treatments can include nonprescription oral decongestants and nasal decongestant sprays, as well as nasal corticosteroid sprays. (For more information on these types of medicines, see Chapter 6.)

REMEMBER

If your child has chronic OME that lasts more than six to eight weeks, your pediatrician may refer them to an ENT for surgery. The most common OME treatment procedures are

>> **Adenoidectomy:** If your child's ET is chronically blocked and your child is older than 3, your physician may recommend removing their adenoids. (Removing the tonsils is no longer an effective or appropriate procedure for treatment of ear problems.)

>> **Myringotomy:** The ENT makes a small incision in the eardrum that permits drainage of the trapped fluid. This procedure is helpful both for diagnostic purposes (to identify infecting organisms) and to relieve the severe pain, pressure, and fever associated with an acute middle ear infection.

>> **Tympanostomy:** This procedure includes surgically inserting small plastic tubes (known as *pressure equalization* or *PE tubes*) in the eardrum to equalize air pressure in the ear and allow drainage of fluid from the middle ear and ET down to the nasopharynx. ENTs usually perform tympanostomies with a general anesthetic, and occasionally with local anesthetic (for older children or adults), as an outpatient procedure. In most cases, doctors recommend that PE tubes remain in place for 6 to 18 months or until they fall out. Children often don't notice the tubes after they've been in place for a while. Generally, children with PE tubes shouldn't go swimming. However, in some cases, an ENT may fit your child with earplugs, making water activities a possibility.

Diagnosing ear infections

SEE YOUR DOCTOR

The first step in diagnosing suspected ear infections usually involves examining your middle ear. Your physician uses an *otoscope* (a tool that shines a light to help examine the ear canal and ear drum) to look for an obvious sign of infection. AOM often appears as a swollen, red, inflamed bulging of the tympanic membrane (eardrum) with poor or no movement. OME can appear as a pink or white, opaque, withdrawn tympanic membrane with poor or no movement.

Other diagnostic procedures for both AOM and OME may include

>> **Audiometry:** This procedure evaluates the effect of chronic middle ear effusions on a person's hearing. Audiometry is especially important for children because hearing loss can cause delayed speech and language development.

>> **Tympanometry:** This procedure measures the eardrum's response at various pressure levels and helps diagnose middle ear effusions and ET dysfunction.

Taking preventive measures

As with sinusitis, one of the most important steps you can take to prevent ear infections, if you also have allergic rhinitis, is to effectively treat your allergies, which includes using the avoidance measures we describe in Chapter 5 and taking the appropriate medications, if necessary, to manage your allergic rhinitis symptoms, as we explain in Chapter 6.

You also need to take the preventive measures we describe in the "Describing Sinusitis" section earlier in chapter to keep your sinuses clear if you have an allergy attack or a cold or other upper respiratory infection.

THE INFO ON NASAL POLYPS

Nasal polyps are soft painless growths in the sinuses that can contribute to nasal congestion and otitis media by obstructing airflow, causing a feeling of stuffiness or blockage in the nose. Although small polyps may not cause noticeable symptoms, larger growths can significantly impact breathing and overall comfort. Nasal congestion caused by polyps may be accompanied by other symptoms like a runny nose, loss of smell, facial pressure, and snoring. In some cases, patients with nasal polyps can experience violent and potentially fatal reactions to aspirin and related drugs such as nonsteroidal anti-inflammatory drugs (NSAIDs), including ibuprofen and naproxen.

Treatment of nasal polyps initially involves the use of nasal corticosteroid spray and if not effective, oral corticosteroids may also be used. Recently, three injectable biologic medications have been approved for patients 18 years and older. These biologics include Dupilumab, Mepolizumab, and Omalizumab, which appear to reduce nasal polyp size and improve both sinus and nasal symptoms. If initial conservative treatment doesn't provide effective relief, your physician may consider surgical removal of the nasal polyps.

3

Approaching Asthma

Chapter **8**

Reviewing Asthma Fundamentals

Accoring to many experts, asthma is now a global epidemic, and its prevalence and severity continue to grow in many parts of the world, including the United States, Western Europe, Australia, and New Zealand. More than 25 million people in the United States alone and more than 330 million globally have some form of asthma. In fact, reports from Canada state that the severity of exacerbations in people with asthma is increasing the number of hospitalizations. Taking care of asthma means taking care of your whole body and we're here to help you discover what asthma is, how to treat and manage it, and how to prevent complications.

This chapter starts with the fundamentals of asthma: what it is and how it affects you. It's helpful to understand the contributing factors of asthma, as well as how to live a full life with this condition.

Understanding Asthma

You or someone you love has just been diagnosed with asthma. Feeling concerned or overwhelmed by this unsettling news is only natural. The good news is that physicians now know more than ever about asthma and its related conditions and how to manage it. The following sections help you develop a basic understanding of how asthma can affect you.

REMEMBER

Asthma is a chronic condition that starts with the immune system and can impact many organs, including the lungs. Many organs can be affected, primarily the lungs. A wide range of triggers can lead to an asthma attack or flare. These triggers include exercise, cold air, a virus, pollution, smoke, and frequently, a host of allergens. In fact, about 80 percent of children with asthma also have identifiable allergies. We talk more about allergies and how they're related to asthma in Chapter 9.

Your lungs and airways are vital to your health. Interestingly, the lungs are the largest internal organ in the body. Laid flat they're roughly the same size as a tennis court. That's indicative of nature's assessment of the importance of this organ. This network of bronchial tubes enables your lungs to absorb oxygen into the blood and also get rid of carbon dioxide. This process is called *respiration* or, more commonly, *breathing.* Most people take breathing for granted unless something interferes with the process by obstructing your airways.

How normal breathing works

To better understand how asthma adversely affects your airways, consider what happens in normal breathing:

1. **The air you inhale flows into your nose and/or mouth and into your** *trachea,* **or windpipe.**

2. **Your trachea then divides in the lung into right and left main** *bronchi,* **or branches, funneling the air into each of your lungs.**

3. **The main bronchi continue branching out into your lungs and dividing into a network of airways called** *bronchial tubes.*

   The exterior of your bronchial tubes consists of layers of muscles. These muscles help to dilate (relax) and constrict (tighten) as you inhale and exhale. Physicians refer to airway relaxation as *bronchodilation* and to the tightening that can help your lungs push out air when you exhale as *bronchoconstriction*.

4. **Your network of airways ultimately leads to the** *alveoli,* **tiny air sacs that look like small clusters of grapes.**

   They contain blood vessels that enable vital respiratory exchange.

5. **Oxygen from the air you breathe is absorbed into the bloodstream, while carbon dioxide gas from your blood exits your body as you exhale.**

In asthma, airway obstruction often occurs as a result of an underlying airway inflammatory reaction that leads to one or more of the following clinical responses:

- Airway hyperresponsiveness

- Airway constriction

- Airway congestion

These inflammatory responses can lead to a vicious cycle in which the airways become increasingly more sensitive and inflamed because they're constantly responding to allergens, irritants, and other factors.

What you can't see can hurt you

If your body were transparent so that you could see what happens internally, it's likely more physicians would treat asthma earlier and more aggressively, because you and your physician would be much more aware of how the underlying disease affects you.

As we explain in the section "Testing your lungs" later in the chapter, you need to make sure that your physician performs appropriate *pulmonary* (lung) function tests (PFTs) if you're experiencing bouts of wheezing, recurring coughs, lingering colds, or other symptoms that may indicate an underlying respiratory condition.

How airway obstruction develops

Here's an overview of how the mechanisms of asthma interact. We itemize these processes to explain them, but keep in mind that they're often ongoing events that can occur simultaneously in your lungs. Figure 8-1 compares a normal airway with that of a patient with asthma.

» **Airway constriction:** When a trigger or precipitating factor irritates your airways, it can cause the release of chemical mediators such as histamine and leukotrienes (see Chapter 2) from the mast cells. These released chemical mediators cause inflammatory responses of the *epithelium* (the lining of the airway), and the muscles around your bronchial tubes can also tighten, leading to *airway constriction*. This process results in narrowing airways and difficulty breathing.

» **Airway hyperresponsiveness:** The underlying airway inflammation in asthma can cause *airway hyperresponsiveness* as the muscles around your bronchial tubes twitch or constrict. This twitchy feeling indicates that your muscles are overreacting/constricting, causing acute bronchoconstriction or bronchospasm. This can occur even if you're exposed to otherwise harmless substances, such as allergens and irritants that rarely provoke reactions in people without asthma and allergies (refer to the section "Revealing the Many Facets of Asthma," later in this chapter).

>> **Airway congestion:** Mucus and fluids are often released as part of the inflammatory process. This can accumulate in your airways, overwhelming the *cilia* (tiny hairlike projections from certain cells that sweep debris-laden mucus through your airways) and leading to *airway congestion.* This accumulation of mucus and fluids may make you feel the urge to cough up phlegm to relieve your chest congestion.

>> **Airway edema:** The long-term release of inflammatory fluids in constricted, hyperresponsive, and congested airways can frequently lead to *airway edema* (swelling of the airway). As a result, bronchial tubes become more rigid, further interfering with airflow. In severe cases of airway congestion and edema, a chronic buildup of mucus secretion leads to the formation of mucus plugs in the airway, which can limit the flow of air in and out of the airways of the lungs.

>> **Airway remodeling:** If airway inflammation is left untreated or poorly managed for many years, the constant injury to your bronchial tubes due to ongoing airway constriction, airway hyperresponsiveness, and airway congestion can lead to *airway remodeling.* As a result, scar tissue can permanently replace your normal airway tissue. With this airway remodeling, airway obstruction can persist and may not respond well to treatment, leading to the eventual loss of airway function and potentially, irreversible lung damage.

>> **Cellular Infiltration:** This complex cellular mechanism, characterized by either predominant eosinophils or neutrophils, is involved in the airway remodeling seen in chronic asthma. As physicians continue to gain a better understanding of this process, improved and innovative therapeutic approaches allow for more targeted treatments of asthma and allergic diseases (see Chapter 6).

REMEMBER

This vicious cycle of asthma can develop gradually, over hours or even days following exposure to triggers or precipitating factors. After this process is set in motion, you can potentially suffer severe and long-lasting consequences.

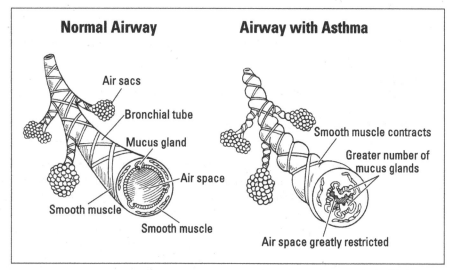

© John Wiley & Sons, Inc.

FIGURE 8-1: A normal airway and an airway with asthma. Note the muscle constriction (bronchospasm) and airway inflammation.

Identifying Who Gets Asthma and Why

The best predictor that an individual may develop asthma is a family history of allergies and asthma and/or *atopy*, an inherited tendency to develop hypersensitivities to allergic triggers. This tendency is almost always due to an overactive immune response that produces elevated levels of immunoglobulin E (IgE) antibodies to allergens. (See Chapter 2 for an extensive discussion of this process.)

Genetic inheritance can be a significant factor in developing this condition. The predisposition of asthma is often seen in other family members. In fact, two-thirds of asthma patients have a family member who also has the disease.

Most cases of asthma are of an allergic nature (known as *allergic asthma*), and usually are first seen during childhood, affecting boys more often than girls. Asthma is the most common chronic disease of childhood. Other indicators of atopy in young children, including allergic disorders, such as food allergies, *atopic dermatitis* (allergic eczema), or *allergic rhinitis* (hay fever), can precede this condition, frequently referred to as *childhood-onset asthma*.

Adult-onset asthma occurs less frequently and develops in adults older than 40, more often in women. Atopy doesn't appear to play a role in these cases. Rather, adult-onset asthma most often seems to be triggered by various nonallergic factors, including sinusitis, upper respiratory infections, nasal polyps, gastroesophageal reflux disease (GERD), sensitivities to aspirin and related nonsteroidal anti-inflammatory drugs (NSAIDs), as well as occupational exposures to chemicals, such as those found in fumes, gases, resins, dust, and insecticides. However, many asthma symptoms seem to occur spontaneously without identifiable triggers.

Keep these points in mind about asthma:

>> Important symptoms of asthma in infancy and early childhood include persistent coughing, wheezing, and recurring or lingering chest colds.

>> Inflammation of the airways is the single most important underlying factor in asthma. If you have asthma, your symptoms may come and go, but the underlying inflammation usually persists. Episodes of asthma symptoms can vary in length from minutes to hours and even from days to weeks, often depending on the severity of your symptoms (see Chapter 10), and the character of the triggering mechanism (see Chapter 9).

>> Although no cure for asthma presently exists, in most cases you can manage and even reverse the effects of the disease. However, poorly managed or undertreated asthma can lead to loss of airway function and, in some cases, irreversible lung damage as a result of airway remodeling. (Read about airway remodeling in the section "How airway obstruction develops" earlier in this chapter.)

>> Early, comprehensive treatment with appropriate medication is vital to effectively manage your asthma.

Effectively managing your asthma also means understanding what triggers your respiratory symptoms and will be discussed in the following sections.

Recognizing triggers, attacks, episodes, and symptoms

A wide variety of allergens, irritants, and other factors, such as colds, flu, exercise, and drug sensitivities, can trigger asthma symptoms what may be referred to as *asthma attacks* or *asthma episodes*. (See Chapter 6 for more information about asthma triggers and how to avoid them.) Asthma symptoms can range from decreased ability to exercise, to feeling completely out of breath, and from persistent coughing to wheezing, chest tightness, or life-threatening respiratory distress. In many cases, a persistent cough may be the only initial presenting symptom of asthma.

WARNING

Experiencing asthma symptoms, whatever the intensity, means that your asthma isn't currently well controlled. Such symptoms may indicate that your asthma needs more effective management, as we explain in the section "Managing Asthma Effectively" later in this chapter.

Accepting that asthma isn't all in your head

In the past, some healthcare providers and family members perceived asthma as a nervous disorder, thought to be caused by anxiety and psychological stress. Physicians and researchers now know that this misconception has no basis in fact. Asthma occurs in the airways of your lungs, not in your head.

Although anxiety and stress can possibly aggravate your asthma (as well as other illnesses), psychological factors don't actually cause your condition. Unfortunately, we still hear stories from friends and family of individuals with asthma who believe that asthma is just "all in the patient's head." They mistakenly insist that if the person would just calm down that their condition would go away. However, instead of stress causing asthma, it's usually the other way around: Breathing problems can cause stress. Stressing out because you can't breathe is a perfectly natural and understandable response.

Therefore, a proper diagnosis of asthma and/or allergies and early, aggressive treatment for these conditions are crucial. In most cases, you should be able to control your asthma and allergic condition so that it doesn't control you, thus enabling you to lead a full and active life. Remember, asthma and allergies can affect anyone: from the captain of the chess team to the captain of the football team as well as everybody in between.

Preventing asthma: Can it be done?

Although totally preventing asthma isn't yet achievable, you and your physician can design a step-by-step plan to effectively control your condition and significantly reduce the risk of future asthma attacks.

TIP

Create a detailed plan with your physician for taking medications and managing an asthma attack and then follow that action plan. (See the section "Being ready with your asthma self-management" later in this chapter.) Careful planning and avoiding asthma triggers are the best ways to prevent asthma attacks, especially in children as their lungs develop.

The following are some proactive steps you should include in your plan:

» **Limit exposure to asthma triggers.** Avoid the allergens and irritants that trigger asthma symptoms.

» **Exercise frequently and encourage your child with asthma to do so too.** As long as your asthma is well controlled, regular physical activity can help your lungs work more efficiently

» **Don't allow smoking around you (or your child).** Exposure to tobacco smoke during infancy is a strong predictive factor for childhood asthma as well as a common trigger of asthma attacks.

» **Maintain a healthy weight.** Being overweight can worsen asthma symptoms, and it increases your risk for other health problems.

» **Keep heartburn under control.** Acid reflux or severe heartburn (GERD) may worsen your asthma symptoms. You may need over-the-counter (OTC) or prescription medications to control your acid reflux.

» **See your physician when necessary.** Check in regularly. Don't ignore signs that your asthma may not be under control, such as needing to use a quick-relief inhaler too often. Asthma changes over time. Consulting your physician can help you make necessary treatment adjustments to keep symptoms under control.

ADDRESSING INEQUITIES IN ASTHMA CARE

According to the Centers for Disease Control and Prevention (CDC), disparities in health-care in the United States are a driving force in the increasing prevalence of asthma. This prevalence is most notable among children and adults of lower socio-economic status, non-Hispanic Black children, and women.

Healthy People 2020 (the federal government's framework for a healthier country) defines health disparities as "a particular type of health difference that is closely linked with social, economic, and/or environmental disadvantage." Social determinants of health, including limited medical care options, economic challenges, substandard housing, lack of transportation, decreased access to medical healthcare specialists, as well as cultural and language barriers, racial discrimination, and polluted environments, may account for much of these disparities. Reducing health disparities and promoting health equity are both priorities of the CDC and Healthy People 2020.

Health equity is defined by the National Library of Medicine as "the state in which everyone has the opportunity to attain full health potential, and no one is disadvantaged from achieving this potential because of social position or any other socially defined circumstance."

Achieving greater health equity in asthma care so that all patients have the best opportunity to lead healthier and more fulfilling lives also requires expanding health literacy, particularly among disadvantaged communities.

Clearly there's an urgent need to improve health literacy and social determinants of health, and to reduce disparities in treatment and outcomes between more affluent and less affluent asthma patients. In response a community-based program, called Not One More Life (NOML) was developed in 2002 to provide education, screening, counseling, and monitoring, bringing asthma care to churches and schools in historically underserved communities. It provides a model for helping asthma patients thrive despite the economic and social hardships they may face. The NOML program is now housed at Allergy & Asthma Network and serves thousands of people each year in underserved communities. For more information on NOML and this topic, please visit `https://allergyasthmanetwork.org/health-disparities/`.

Revealing the Many Facets of Asthma

Asthma can appear in many different ways. The underlying mechanism causing many of the symptoms of asthma is due to a complex series of events involving several types of cells and tissues that reside in your lungs.

A wide range of factors can cause asthma symptoms, and because certain triggers can result in stronger reactions in some asthma patients than in others, physicians often classify asthma according to these triggers. Classifying asthma in this way can help you and your physician better understand what's causing your symptoms.

Although a certain precipitating factor may predominate in many asthma cases, multiple triggers affect the majority of people with asthma. For example, most asthma patients have exercise-induced asthma, sometimes known as exercise-induced bronchospasm — which we explain in the "Exercise-induced asthma (EIA)" later in this section — in addition to asthma that manifests from other triggers or precipitating factors. The next sections list the main asthma classifications that many physicians use.

Allergic asthma

Allergic (or *atopic*) asthma is a type of asthma that's triggered by allergens like pollens, pets, and dust mites. The vast majority of people with allergic asthma have a related condition such as *allergic rhinitis* (hay fever), *atopic dermatitis* (eczema), or food allergies.

If you have allergic asthma, your physician is likely to prescribe a *preventer inhaler* to take on a regular basis and a *reliever inhaler* to use only when you have asthma symptoms. Needless to say, it's also important to avoid your asthma triggers as much as possible.

Nonallergic asthma

Nonallergic asthma, or *nonatopic* asthma, is a type of asthma that isn't related to a particular allergy trigger like pollen or dust and is less commonly seen than allergic asthma. The causes aren't well understood, but it often develops later in life (older than 40) and is often more severe than other types of asthma.

Occupational asthma

Occupational asthma is caused directly by your work environment. You may have occupational asthma if

>> Your asthma symptoms started in adulthood.

>> Your asthma symptoms improve on the days you're not at work.

Occupational asthma is usually a type of allergic asthma. For example, if you work in a bakery, you may be allergic to flour dust, or if you work in a healthcare environment, the dust from latex gloves can trigger your symptoms.

REMEMBER

If you think you may have occupational asthma, make an appointment to see your healthcare provider so you can get the right diagnosis and appropriate treatment.

Exercise-induced asthma (EIA)

Some people without a confirmed diagnosis of asthma can experience asthma-like symptoms triggered only by exercise. This is often called *exercise-induced asthma* (EIA), but a better term is *exercise-induced bronchoconstriction* (EIB) because the tightening and narrowing of the airways (bronchoconstriction) isn't caused by pre-existing asthma. EIB commonly affects elite athletes or people doing strenuous exercise in very cold conditions.

If you don't have a diagnosis of asthma but you're experiencing symptoms such as chest tightness, breathlessness, coughing, or fatigue during or after exercising, ask your healthcare provider to do the following:

>> **Test your lung function with a spirometry test.** This is to make sure you don't have underlying asthma. Refer to the "Testing your lungs" section later in this chapter.

>> **Do an exercise challenge test.** Usually done on a treadmill or other equipment, this is a way to see how your airways react to exercise. Spirometry tests before and after your exercise test can determine whether you have EIB by observing a decrease in your lung function after physical exertion.

>> **Prescribe treatments to help with the symptoms you're experiencing so you can continue to exercise safely.** This may be a reliever inhaler to take immediately before you exercise.

If you need to use your pre-exercise reliever inhaler daily to stop exercise symptoms from developing, or three or more times a week to relieve symptoms, you should consider changing to a different treatment regimen. Your physician may suggest using a daily preventer inhaler or add-on treatments like montelukast (Singulair) or long-acting bronchodilators.

Aspirin-induced asthma (AIA)

Aspirin-induced asthma (AIA) is a condition in which asthma symptoms can be triggered by taking aspirin or other NSAIDs. It's more commonly known as *aspirin-exacerbated respiratory disease* (AERD) or Samter's Triad. The American Academy of Allergy, Asthma, & Immunology (AAAAI) estimates that 9 percent of adults have asthma and about one-third of these adults who have asthma and nasal polyps may also have AERD.

Acetylsalicylic acid (aspirin) is a type of NSAID used to relieve pain, inflammation, and fever. Similar medications include ibuprofen (Advil, Motrin) and naproxen (Aleve).

Aspirin and other NSAIDs interact with an enzyme known as cyclooxygenase-1 (COX-1). Although the exact triggers are unknown, it's thought that people with AERD have a sensitivity to the way these medications inhibit COX-1.

You may be more prone to AERD if you have all three of these conditions:

>> Asthma

>> Chronic sinusitis

>> Nasal polyps

A physician may still recommend aspirin for the treatment of other conditions, such as preventing heart attacks or strokes, in cases where a person may have already experienced one of these conditions.

Food allergies and food-induced anaphylaxis

For some people, there may be an indirect connection between food and asthma. Although food isn't a common asthma trigger, your asthma can be affected by eating. Asthma can also affect how you react if you have food allergies.

Although very rare, some people may notice certain foods affect their asthma. High amounts of *sulfites,* a type of preservative used in foods, may trigger asthma in these individuals. Foods that are high in sulfites may include wine, beer, and pickled foods.

If your healthcare provider has diagnosed a food allergy, then avoiding the food(s) that trigger your reactions is the best way to prevent problems. Visit Kids With Food Allergies for more information that applies to children as well as adults: https://kidswithfoodallergies.org/what-is-anaphylaxis

WARNING

Mild and severe symptoms of food allergies can progress to a life-threatening allergic reaction called *anaphylaxis* (anna-fih-*lack*-sis). This reaction usually involves more than one part of the body and can deteriorate quickly. Anaphylaxis must be treated immediately to provide the best chance to resolve the symptoms and prevent serious complications.

A severe food allergic reaction can cause trouble breathing. It may be hard to know if you're having a food allergic reaction or an asthma attack. Here are some ways to tell the difference:

>> If you're only coughing, wheezing, or having trouble breathing and don't have any symptoms involving other parts of your body, it's probably asthma. Follow your asthma action plan.

>> If you had asthma symptoms before eating the food, it's probably asthma. Follow your asthma action plan.

>> Food allergy symptoms, like itchy lips or mouth, usually develop quickly after you eat the food to which you're allergic. Follow your food allergy plan.

>> Severe allergic reactions involve two or more body systems. An allergic reaction may involve breathing difficulties, hives, swelling, itchy mouth and throat, nausea, or vomiting. Follow your anaphylaxis action plan (see the next list).

REMEMBER

If you have a food allergy, remember these vital points:

» Some severe allergic food reactions require a second dose of epinephrine to be administered. Always carry two prescribed epinephrine auto-injectors or intranasal epinephrine with you.

» Ask your physician to help you create an anaphylaxis action plan, which instructs you on what to do if you have a severe reaction. You can find a sample plan on the Kids with Food Allergies website at https://kidswithfoodallergies.org/what-is-anaphylaxis.

» Train trusted friends, family, and coworkers on how to use an epinephrine auto-injector or intranasal epinephrine in an emergency and have them practice regularly.

» If you're having difficulty breathing and aren't sure if you're having an allergic reaction or an asthma attack, treat it like a food allergic reaction and use your epinephrine auto-injector or intranasal epinephrine.

Diagnosing Asthma

Effectively managing your asthma starts with your physician correctly diagnosing your condition. To determine whether asthma causes your respiratory symptoms, your physician should take your medical history, perform a physical exam, test your lung function, and perform other tests, as we explain in the following sections.

REMEMBER

Asthma symptoms vary widely from patient to patient. In fact, your own symptoms may change over time. Make sure your physician establishes these key points when diagnosing your asthma:

» You experience symptoms of airway obstruction.

» Your airway obstruction is at least partially reversible (and responds well to treatment).

» Your symptoms clearly result from asthma, not from other conditions that we describe in "Diagnosing other possible disorders" later in this chapter.

Taking your medical history

A careful, thorough medical history is the first step in diagnosing the correct cause of your respiratory symptoms. For this reason, your physician may ask several questions about your condition and your activities. Keeping track of symptoms in a diary may help you provide your physician with details that can assist in making the proper diagnosis. Try to provide as much information as possible concerning the following topics:

>> The type of symptoms you experience, which may include coughing, wheezing, shortness of breath, chest tightness, and *productive coughs* (coughs that bring up mucus).

>> The pattern of your symptoms:

- *Perennial* (year-round), seasonal, or perennial with seasonal worsening.

- Constant, *episodic* (occasional), or constant with episodic worsening.

>> The onset of your symptoms. At what rate do your symptoms develop — rapidly or slowly? And can that rate vary?

>> The duration and frequency of your symptoms and whether the type and intensity of symptoms vary at different times of day and night. Especially note if your episodes awaken you from sleep or are more severe when you wake up in the morning.

>> The impact that exercise or other physical exertion has on your symptoms.

>> Your exposure to potential asthma triggers. In addition to the allergens, irritants, and precipitating factors listed in the section "Revealing the Many Facets of Asthma" earlier in this chapter, your physician needs to be informed about hormonal factors, such as adrenal or thyroid disease. Special considerations for women are pregnancy or changes in their menstrual cycles.

>> The progression of your disease, including any treatment and medications you've received or taken and their effectiveness. Your physician especially wants to know whether you presently take or have previously taken oral corticosteroids (for example, prednisone) and, if so, the dosage and the frequency of use of this medication.

>> Your family history, especially whether parents, siblings, or close relatives suffer from asthma, allergic or nonallergic rhinitis, and other types of allergies, sinusitis, or nasal polyps.

>> Your lifestyle, including

- Your home environment, such as its age and location; type of cooling and heating system; your basement's condition; whether you have a wood-burning stove, humidifier, carpet and padding, or mold and mildew; and the types of bedding, carpeting, and furniture coverings you use.

- Whether anyone smokes in your home or the other locations where you spend time, such as work or school.

- Any history of substance abuse.

>> The impact of the disease on you and your family, such as

- Any life-threatening symptoms, emergency or urgent care treatments, or hospitalizations.

- The number of days you (or your child with asthma) have missed from school or work, the disease's economic impact, and its effect on your recreational activities.

- If your child has asthma, your physician may ask you about the effects of the illness on your youngster's growth, development, behavior, and ability to participate in sports.

>> Your knowledge, perception, and beliefs about asthma and long-term management of the disease, as well as your ability to cope with the illness.

>> The level of support and assistance you receive from your family members and their abilities to recognize a sudden worsening of your symptoms.

Examining your physical condition

A physical exam for suspected asthma usually focuses not only on your breathing passageways but also on other characteristics and symptoms of atopic disease. The significant physical signs of asthma or allergy that your physician looks for primarily include the following:

>> Chest deformity, such as an expanded or overinflated chest, as well as hunched shoulders

>> Coughing, wheezing, shortness of breath, and other respiratory symptoms

>> Increased nasal discharge, swelling, and the presence of nasal polyps

>> Signs of sinus disease, such as thick or discolored nasal discharge

>> Any allergic skin conditions, such as eczema — refer to the section "Identifying Who Gets Asthma and Why" earlier in this chapter

Testing your lungs

Many people are used to routinely taking their temperature or regularly having their physician check their pulse and blood pressure, in addition to monitoring their blood sugar and cholesterol levels on a consistent basis. However, most people aren't having appropriate *pulmonary* (lung) function tests, which may be why asthma is so frequently not diagnosed at an early stage but rather, only after a severe episode.

Objective pulmonary function tests are the most reliable means of assessing the extent to which your lung function is limited or affected. The following sections explain the most important tests that physicians most often use to diagnose asthma. (See Chapter 10 for a more detailed description of these tests.)

Spirometry

To determine if you have airway obstruction and whether your condition is *reversible* (can improve with appropriate treatment), physicians often use a *spirometer* to measure the volume of air you exhale from your large and small airways before and 15 minutes after inhaling a short-acting beta$_2$-adrenergic bronchodilator. Figure 8-2 shows a patient using a spirometer.

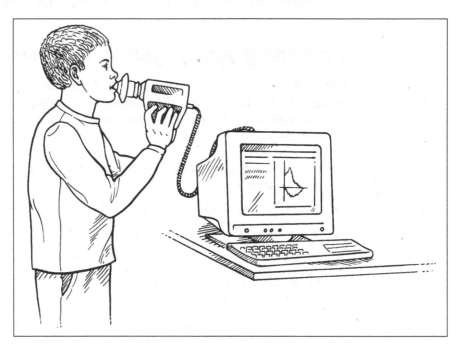

FIGURE 8-2:
A spirometer measures airflow.

Spirometry provides many types of airflow measurements, including the following:

>> **Forced vital capacity (FVC):** The maximum volume (in liters) of air you can exhale after taking in the deepest breath you can manage.

>> **Forced expiratory volume (FEV1):** The volume (in liters) of air you're able to exhale when you breathe out with maximal effort in the first second, as forcefully as possible. Physicians determine a reduction in FEV1 as the most common indicator of airway obstruction in patients with symptoms of asthma. This test, the most important measurement in the diagnosis and management of asthma, generally measures obstruction of the large airways, although FEV1 can also reveal severe obstruction of the small airways. A baseline FEV1 (before using a bronchodilator) that's lower than normal but increases by at least 12 percent 15 minutes after you inhale a short-acting bronchodilator (post-bronchodilator) allows your physician to conclusively establish the diagnosis of asthma.

>> **Maximum midexpiratory flow (MMEF):** The middle part of your forced exhalation (in liters per second). This measurement is also referred to as the *forced expiratory flow between 25 and 75 percent* (FEF 25–75 percent) of FVC. A reduction in MMEF can indicate obstruction of the lungs' small airways.

Your physician compares the values from the spirometry to the predicted normal reference values, based on your age, height, sex, and race, as established by the American Thoracic Society. The percent of the predicted normal value of your measured FEV1 is one of the major criteria that your physician uses to classify your level of asthma severity. (See Chapter 10 for information on the four levels of asthma severity.)

Physicians consider spirometry a valuable tool for diagnosing childhood cases of asthma in patients older than 4 years. However, for younger children, the test can be difficult, if not impossible, to perform. In those cases, your child's physician may decide that trying a peak-flow meter or another less complicated assessment process is more suitable.

Although spirometry is the most common and widely used lung function test, another test called DLCO (diffusing capacity of the lungs for carbon monoxide) is a measurement used by physicians to assess the lung's ability to transfer gas from expired air into the bloodstream. This measurement is often used to differentiate asthma from chronic obstructive pulmonary disease (COPD).

Impulse oscillometry (IOS)

Impulse oscillometry (IOS) is a pulmonary function test that, unlike spirometry, isn't effort dependent and measures total airway resistance. IOS has advantages over spirometry because it's easier to perform on young children in the diagnosis and assessment of asthma. It has been effectively used in children as young as 3 years of age.

Peak-flow meters

Peak-flow meters, which are available in a variety of shapes and sizes from different manufacturers, are convenient, portable, and easy-to-use devices for monitoring *peak expiratory flow rate* (PEFR), the maximum rate of air (in liters per minute) you can force out of your large airways, as a measurement of lung function. This measurement isn't as accurate as spirometry, but you can easily perform it at home. Measurements of PEFR are also a vital part of long-term management of your asthma, as we explain in more depth in Chapter 10.

Challenge tests

If spirometry indicates normal or near-normal lung functions but asthma continues to seem the most likely cause of your symptoms, your physician may decide that a form of challenge test is indicated for a more conclusive diagnosis.

Challenge tests, also called *bronchoprovocation,* usually involve your physician administering small doses of inhaled methacholine or histamine, or making you exercise under observation. The goal of these tests is to see whether the challenges cause obstructive changes in your airways, thus provoking mild asthma symptoms. Your physician usually measures your lung functions before and after each test.

Diagnosing other possible disorders

REMEMBER

Although asthma causes most recurring episodes of coughing, wheezing, and shortness of breath, other disorders can cause these symptoms in some cases. With infants and children, underlying problems may include

>> An upper respiratory disease, such as allergic rhinitis or sinusitis

>> A swallowing mechanism problem or the effects of GERD

>> Congenital heart disease, often leading to congestive heart failure

>> An obstruction of large airways, possibly caused by

- A foreign object in the trachea or main bronchi, such as a small piece of popcorn your child may have accidentally inhaled.

- Problems of the *larynx* (the cartilaginous portion of the upper respiratory tract that contains the vocal cords) or with the vocal cords themselves.

- *Tracheal stenosis* is an abnormal narrowing of the *trachea* (windpipe) that restricts your ability to breathe normally. This condition is sometimes referred to as *subglottic stenosis.*
- Benign or malignant tumors or enlarged lymph nodes.

>> An obstruction of the small airways, as a result of

- Cystic fibrosis
- Abnormal development of the bronchi and lungs
- Viral infection of the *bronchioles* (small bronchi)

With adult cases, underlying problems may include

>> Chronic bronchitis and/or emphysema, collectively referred to as COPD

>> *Pulmonary embolism* (a blood clot, air bubble, bacterial mass, or other mass that can clog a blood vessel)

>> Heart disease

>> Problems of the vocal cords or the larynx (vocal cord dysfunction, paradoxical vocal fold motion disorder)

>> Benign or malignant tumors in the airways

>> A cough reaction due to drugs that you may be using to treat other conditions, such as ACE inhibitors for hypertension

>> In addition, a variety of conditions can be confused with asthma, such as fibrotic lung disease, sarcoid, and eosinophilic alveolitis

Classifying asthma severity

If your physician diagnoses you with asthma based on your medical history, a physical exam, and appropriate tests, studies, and assessments, they also need to define your condition's severity. Physicians classify asthma — whether it's allergic or nonallergic — according to four levels of severity.

Experts have developed these severity classifications, which provide the basis for *stepwise management* of asthma. We explain stepwise management and asthma severity levels in detail in Chapter 10.

Consulting a specialist for diagnosis

To diagnose your condition, you or your physician should consider consulting an asthma specialist, such as an allergist or *pulmonologist* (lung physician), when

>> Your diagnosis is difficult to establish.

>> Your diagnosis requires specialized testing, such as allergy testing (see Chapter 3), bronchoprovocation (see the section "Testing your lungs," earlier in this chapter), or *bronchoscopy* (an exam of the interior of your bronchi using a slender, flexible fiber-optic bronchoscope).

>> Your physician advises you to consider allergy shots (see Chapter 4).

>> Other conditions, such as sinusitis, nasal polyps, severe rhinitis, GERD, COPD, vocal cord problems, or *aspergillosis* (a fungal infection that can affect the lungs), complicate your condition or diagnosis.

>> Your asthma symptoms aren't improving under your present treatment or are actually getting worse.

>> You aren't able to regularly sleep through the night without being awakened by your asthma symptoms.

>> You can't exercise as you'd like to because of asthma.

>> You need to use an asthma inhaler for quick relief on a daily basis or in the middle of the night.

>> You've experienced a previous emergency room visit or hospitalization for asthma (see Chapter 10) or anaphylaxis (see the section "Food allergies and food-induced anaphylaxis" earlier in this chapter).

Managing Asthma Effectively

"Where do I begin?" That's a question many people with asthma ask themselves. For some people, the question may come up as soon as they receive their diagnosis. For other people, the question may arise after they notice complications of their asthma. Still others may face that question as they care for a loved one living with asthma. It's not easy to know how to start taking care of yourself and managing your asthma.

We're here to help point you in the right direction and begin taking better care of yourself. In this section, you discover why it's important to take care of your asthma daily and on an ongoing basis. You also find out about the basics of managing your disease. You're responsible for making healthy choices each day. You make choices about food, exercise, medications, and even seeing your physician. So, it's time to get started!

Being ready with your asthma self-management

You may have heard the terms *asthma self-management plan* or *asthma action plan*. Both terms refer to how you take care of or manage your asthma. Your plan is based on your goals that are achieved through shared decision making with your physician. It's vital to understand that asthma management is no small endeavor. You're the person most responsible for taking care of your asthma 24 hours a day, 7 days a week, 365 days a year. You can take comfort in knowing that many people just like you are figuring out how to manage their asthma, take new medications, and improve their quality of life.

Taking care of yourself

Making yourself a top priority is one of the best ways to manage asthma. After all, only you can truly manage your disease! Start taking care of your asthma so you can feel better most days and so that you feel empowered to effectively manage your condition.

Perhaps leading up to your diagnosis you didn't feel so great. You may have experienced symptoms such as shortness of breath or coughing during sleep. Perhaps you were irritable or out of sorts more than usual. In some ways, it may have felt like a relief to discover a cause for these issues. In other ways, it may have felt scary to find out that asthma was the diagnosis.

The good news is you can feel great living with asthma most of the time. Even if every day isn't a home run, most of the time you can live your life to the fullest. That's because taking care of yourself and managing your asthma can positively impact your daily life. Remember, exercise is a mood booster. It can reduce stress, lessen symptoms of depression, and release those amazing brain chemicals, known as *endorphins,* that make you feel better. Strive to do your best and enjoy the rewards of your efforts.

IN THIS CHAPTER

» **Identifying what's causing your asthma symptoms**

» **Avoiding inhalant allergens**

» **Focusing on exposures in your home**

» **Recognizing triggers in your workplace**

» **Steering clear of food and drug triggers**

» **Dealing with other conditions that can aggravate your asthma**

Chapter **9**

Recognizing Asthma Triggers

A voiding or limiting your exposure to factors that bring on your asthma symptoms is vital for managing your condition. Steering clear of asthma triggers can help you experience fewer respiratory symptoms and potentially allow you to reduce your need for medication, especially rescue drugs such as short-acting beta$_2$-adrenergic (beta$_2$-agonist) bronchodilators. (See Dr. Berger's book *Asthma For Dummies* [John Wiley & Sons, Inc.] for details on asthma medications.) Controlling your condition often requires dealing with a host of precipitating factors — a particularly familiar situation if you have allergic asthma, one of the most common types of asthma. Allergic asthma is usually associated with *allergic rhinitis* (hay fever) and/or *allergic conjunctivitis* (red, itchy, watery eyes due to allergens; see Chapter 8 for details about allergic asthma).

Throughout this chapter, we provide information and tips, based on extensive experience and the latest research findings, that can help you — in shared decision-making with your physician — take practical and effective measures to avoid or reduce exposure to your asthma triggers.

Identifying Asthma Triggers

All people with asthma have what we describe as increased bronchial activity. This means their *bronchi* (airways in the lungs) are *hyperactive* in that they respond to exposure to inhaled substances in an exaggerated manner. These bronchi often react at lower doses of the substance (irritant or allergen), and their reactions are more intense than the responses of normal bronchi. This bronchial hyperactivity is central to the disease and can be used to distinguish people with asthma from those who don't have asthma. In addition, a strong correlation exists between the degree of bronchial hyperactivity and the overall severity of a given case. Anything that increases this hyperactivity makes asthma worse and treatments that diminish this hyperactivity can make asthma better.

When we talk about triggers, distinguishing triggers that can increase bronchial hyperactivity from those that don't is essential. Those that worsen hyperactivity do so by producing an inflammatory response in the bronchial tubes. Because of this inflammatory reaction, worsening of the disease for long periods of time, even after the trigger has been removed, can occur. Bronchial hyperactivity also predisposes a person to lung scarring and remodeling. Exercise typically doesn't worsen airway hyperactivity. This is why physicians frequently use only albuterol without an anti-inflammatory medication to treat exercise-induced asthma. On the other hand, allergen exposure can cause a prolonged increase in bronchial hyperactivity. A single exposure to an allergen, a cat, for example, can even increase hyperactivity for several days and even weeks.

The next sections outline allergic and nonallergic triggers that often adversely affect people with asthma.

Evaluating triggers

REMEMBER

One of the most important steps you can take to effectively manage your asthma is to identify what triggers the symptoms of your condition. These triggers (see Figure 9-1) include

» Inhalant allergens, such as animal dander, dust mite and cockroach allergens, some mold spores, and certain airborne grass, weed, and tree pollens (see Chapter 5).

» Irritants and allergens found primarily in the workplace that induce occupational asthma (see "Minimizing Workplace Exposures," later in this chapter) or aggravate an already existing form of the disease.

» Other irritants that you inhale, such as tobacco smoke, household cleaning products, and indoor and outdoor air pollution.

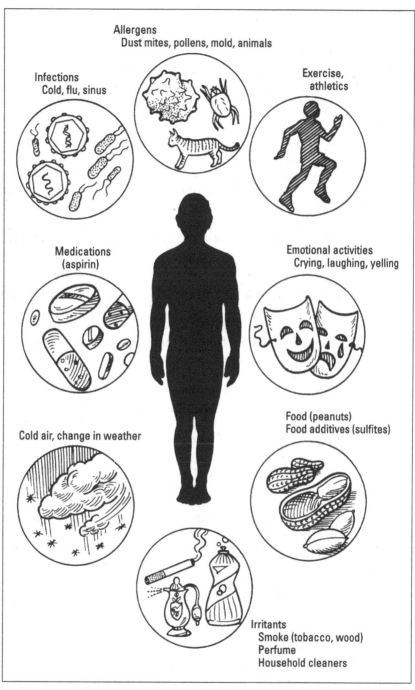

FIGURE 9-1:
Common asthma triggers.

© John Wiley & Sons, Inc

>> Nonallergic triggers, including exercise and physical stimuli such as variations in air temperature and humidity levels.

>> Other medical conditions, including *rhinitis* (stuffy nose), *sinusitis* (sinus infection), gastroesophageal reflux disease (GERD), and viral infections; sensitivities to aspirin, beta-blockers, and other drugs; and sensitivities to particular food additives.

>> Emotional responses, such as crying, laughing, or even yelling. Although emotions aren't the direct triggers of asthma symptoms — and clearly asthma isn't an "emotional problem" — responses associated with strong emotions can induce coughing or wheezing in people with preexisting hyperreactive airways (see Chapter 8), as well as in individuals who don't have asthma but may suffer from other respiratory disorders. For example, your friend with a bad cold may say, "Please don't make me laugh; if I do, I'll start coughing."

Tracking and testing for allergic triggers

To determine what triggers your asthma symptoms and your sensitivity levels to those triggers, your physician should take a thorough medical history. You can assist in this assessment by keeping an asthma diary (see Chapter 3).

Many asthma patients experience *perennial* (year-round) symptoms that worsen during particular seasons. Because a wide range of triggers can contribute to perennial asthma episodes, it is helpful to provide your physician with a record of the seasonal patterns of your symptoms.

For example, if your asthma consistently worsens during late summer and fall in the eastern parts of the United States, your physician may suspect ragweed or mold as a primary cause of the allergic reactions that aggravate your condition. However, physicians usually advise allergy testing (see Chapter 4 for a complete explanation of allergy testing) to investigate possible causes and to confirm the diagnosis and determine appropriate treatment.

TIP

If you have persistent asthma (see Chapter 8) with year-round symptoms that occur primarily indoors, allergy testing can help your doctor identify several of the triggers, such as dust mites, that may be affecting you.

Nocturnal or *nighttime asthma* — which often shows up as a cough, wheezing, or shortness of breath that disturbs your sleep and may require you to use your short-acting adrenergic bronchodilator (see Dr. Berger's book *Asthma For Dummies* [John Wiley & Sons, Inc.] for more information) — can often be severe. Almost all patients with asthma have worsening symptoms at night; in other words, noctur-nal symptoms are *intrinsic* to the disease. Although we aren't sure what the underlying cause of worsening nighttime symptoms is, we think an important cause is the variation in body functions known as the circadian rhythm. The *circadian rhythm* (also known as *diurnal variation*) controls your body's internal clock and may affect your asthma by making you more susceptible to symptoms in the early morning hours (around 3 to 5 a.m.). Also, during the late evening and early morning hours, a number of changes in hormone levels can affect asthma. These include a decrease in plasma levels of hormones from the *adrenal glands* (glands above your kidneys), perhaps the most important of which is *cortisol*. At the same time, a decrease in plasma epinephrine and an increase in plasma histamine also occur.

Allergens in your bedroom, postnasal drip from allergic rhinitis (see Chapter 6), or chronic sinus problems such as sinusitis (see Chapter 7) often trigger nocturnal asthma. Other factors that can cause nocturnal asthma include

>> GERD

>> Airway cooling and drying

>> Lying down in bed (instead of sitting)

>> A bi-phasic response, which includes the immediate reaction and a delayed reaction known as a *late-phase reaction* to allergens you've been exposed to during the day

Reducing Exposure to Inhalant Allergens

Inhalant allergen triggers, also known as *aeroallergens*, are probably the most familiar asthma precipitants because they're also associated with allergic rhinitis and similar conditions (see Chapter 7). If you have allergic asthma, reducing your exposure to inhalant allergens is an important step to take — in shared decision-making with your physician — to manage your condition.

The following sections detail the most common inhalant allergens to look out for.

Animal allergens

Pet dander, which may contain traces of saliva, is a potent trigger of symptoms for many people with asthma. Although household dogs and cats are the most common sources of these allergens, all warm-blooded animals, such as horses, rabbits, small rodents, and birds, produce dander — regardless of their hair length (the source of the allergen is actually the skin rather than the hair). Urine from these animals is another source of allergens. Animal dander also serves as a food supply (along with dead human skin cells) for dust mites, as we explain in Chapter 7.

Dust mites

Dust mites exist almost everywhere humans settle, and they thrive in mattresses, carpets, upholstered furniture, bed covers, linens, clothes, and plush toys (like stuffed animals). Although completely eliminating these dusty creatures is virtually impossible, you can take practical and effective steps to minimize your exposure to the allergens dust mites produce.

See Chapter 7 for more dirt on dust mites, and Chapter 4 for details on measures to control these allergens.

Cockroaches

As if you need another reason to avoid cockroaches, exposure to allergens from cockroach droppings (yuck!) in house dust can trigger and aggravate your asthma symptoms.

Many patients with asthma being seen in inner-city clinics, which are often in areas with large numbers of cockroaches, have tested positive for cockroach allergens (through allergy skin testing) and have improved after immuno-therapy (allergy shots) with cockroach allergen extract. (See Dr. Berger's book *Asthma For Dummies* [John Wiley & Sons, Inc.] for more information on allergy immunotherapy.)

TIP

To control cockroach allergens in your home, consider taking these key steps:

>> Exterminate cockroach infestations. During the fumigation process, stay out of your home and allow it to air out for several hours before reentering. (This advice applies to anyone, regardless of whether you have asthma.)

>> Clean your entire home thoroughly after extermination.

>> Set roach traps.

>> Seal any cracks in your home to prevent reinfestation.

>> Keep your kitchen clean by washing dishes and cookware promptly and by emptying garbage and recycling containers (including old newspapers) often. Avoid leaving food out.

Mold

The airborne spores that molds (fungal growth) release in typically damp areas of many homes, particularly basements, bathrooms, air conditioners, garbage containers, and carpeting, can trigger allergy and asthma symptoms when you inhale them. Mold can also thrive in leaf piles, compost heaps, cut grass, fertilizer, hay, and barns. Airborne mold spores are more numerous than pollen grains and don't have a limited season. Depending on where you live, you may be exposed to airborne mold spores throughout the year, based on humidity levels.

See Chapter 5 for more moldy matters, including tips on translating mold counts and what you can do to reduce mold exposures.

Pollen

From spring through fall, many varieties of trees, grasses, and weeds release pollen that can trigger symptoms of allergic rhinitis or allergic conjunctivitis. These reactions can also affect your allergic asthma, aggravating the underlying airway inflammation.

Many people primarily associate pollen with outdoor exposure. However, because most pollens are windborne, they can often make their way indoors and trigger your allergy and asthma symptoms in your home.

See Chapter 5 for more pollen particulars, including tips on pollen counts and steps you can take to avoid excessive exposure to pollen, especially during periods of high pollination.

Clearing the Air at Home

Indoor environments at home, work, and school and in cars as well as other enclosed means of transportation can often provide significantly more sources of asthma triggers than the outdoors because most enclosures concentrate irritants and allergens. Therefore, take the time to discover the ways indoor air pollution can induce or aggravate your allergies and asthma, while also working to rid your home of anything that triggers your symptoms.

The following section provides information on allergens and irritants that often contribute to indoor air pollution and can trigger asthma symptoms.

Household irritants

The most significant irritant triggers of asthma in many households are

>> Tobacco smoke (see the next section)

>> Fumes and scents from household cleaners, strongly scented soaps, candles, perfumes, glues, and aerosols

>> Smoke from wood-burning appliances or fireplaces

>> Fumes from unvented gas, oil, or kerosene stoves

Other sources of indoor air pollution include pollens and mold spores that get inside, especially on windy days when windows and doors are open. These allergenic materials can also invade your home via your clothing and hair. In fact, if you have allergic asthma, you may wake up congested and wheezing in the morning because allergenic materials find their way into your house so easily. (The pollen or mold spores in your hair probably wound up on your pillow, so you spent the night breathing those allergens into your nose and lungs.)

We recommend that patients shower and wash their hair before bed when pollen and mold counts are high, especially if they've spent a significant amount of time outdoors that day.

No smoking, please

As far as truly irritating irritants go, tobacco smoke is the number one indoor air pollutant. Secondhand smoke has been associated with an increase in the following adverse health effects:

>> Earlier onset of respiratory allergies

>> Persistent wheezing associated with asthma

>> Decreased lung function

>> Hospital admissions for respiratory infections

>> Increased incidence of *otitis media with effusion,* or inflammation of the middle ear

Tobacco smoke frequently provokes asthma symptoms in children. In fact, numerous studies show that parental smoking, especially by the mother, is a major risk factor in the development of asthma in infants who are exposed to secondhand smoke during the first few months of life. Therefore, don't smoke and make sure the people around you don't smoke, especially if you have children.

Fortunately, due to the increased awareness of the dangers of smoking, the incidence has significantly decreased throughout the United States.

Filters and air-cleaning devices

REMEMBER

The quality of the air you breathe indoors largely depends on the condition of your heating, ventilation, and air-conditioning (HVAC) system, as well as the air and particles that circulate throughout it.

TIP

If you're exposed to airborne allergens and irritants such as animal dander, mold spores, pollen, and tobacco smoke, consider using air filters on your HVAC ducts to reduce the level of allergy and asthma triggers circulating through your home. Keep in mind, however, that these filters don't remove substances that have already settled in bedding, carpeting, and furniture — especially dust mite allergens. Dust mite allergens are generally larger than other airborne allergens and irritants, and they usually fall from the air within a few minutes after being stirred up in dust or air currents.

Physicians often recommend these two types of air filtration systems to reduce indoor levels of airborne allergens and irritants:

>> **High-efficiency particulate arrester (HEPA):** These filters are designed to absorb and contain 99.97 percent of all particles larger than 0.3 microns (1/300 the width of a human hair). If the unit truly operates at that level, only 3 out of 10,000 particles get into your indoor environment. Vacuum cleaners and air purifiers with HEPA and ULPA filters (see the next bullet for more information) can play a vital part in allergy-proofing your home.

>> **Ultra-low particulate air (ULPA):** This system filters more thoroughly than the HEPA process and is designed to absorb and contain 99.99 percent of all particles larger than 0.12 microns.

TIP

If your home doesn't have a central HVAC system, you can purchase stand-alone HEPA and ULPA air cleaners for use in individual rooms.

Vacuum cleaning is also vital for reducing your exposure to allergens and irritants at home. However, many standard vacuum cleaners absorb only larger particles, and they allow many allergens to escape in the exhaust. That's why you may often experience asthma symptoms after doing housework: The vacuuming may have made matters worse for you by simply stirring up triggering substances that you then inhaled.

TIP

To avoid stirring up asthma triggers when you vacuum, ask your physician whether they think investing in a vacuum cleaner that uses a HEPA or ULPA filtration process may work for you. Wearing a facemask while vacuuming can also help limit your exposure to asthma triggers in the air.

Minimizing Workplace Exposures

Exposures to many types of chemicals and dust in workplace environments can induce different forms of occupational asthma. In many cases, people who have asthma but haven't yet developed obvious symptoms of the disease may experience asthma episodes for the first time because of exposure to occupational triggers. Allergic and nonallergic triggers can play a part in occupational asthma, which may account for as many as 15 percent of all new asthma cases each year in the United States.

This section helps you identify common workplace triggers and how to diagnose and treat them.

Targeting workplace triggers

Physicians and other healthcare professionals typically associate occupational asthma with exposure to the following workplace triggers:

» **Industrial irritants:** These irritants can include chemicals, fumes, gases, aerosols, paints, smoke, and other substances you primarily find in the workplace. Tobacco smoke in the workplace has often caused many asthma symptoms. Other irritants in the workplace may include food odors and even heavily scented perfumes and colognes that some coworkers might use.

» **Occupational allergens:** Many jobs involve exposure to or contact with substances made of plant materials, food products, and other items that contain allergenic extracts that can trigger allergic reactions, thus inducing occupational asthma in sensitized people. For example, *Baker's asthma* can occur in workers who have constant respiratory exposure to the allergens contained in flour. (Eating the resulting baked food usually doesn't produce symptoms in these workers, however.) Latex is another common occupational allergen, as we explain in the nearby sidebar.

» **Physical stimuli:** These stimuli include environmental conditions in your workplace, especially variations in temperature and humidity, such as heat and cold extremes or air that's especially dry or humid.

Diagnosing and treating workplace triggers

Diagnosing your occupational asthma is important for your long-term health and the successful management of your disease. The sooner you can effectively avoid or reduce your exposure to triggers at work, the better you can control your asthma.

In diagnosing a case of occupational asthma, your physician may first need to assess the following factors:

>> **The pattern of your symptoms:** Symptoms that improve when you're away from work strongly suggest that your problem is indeed work-related.

>> **Your coworkers' symptoms:** Do your coworkers suffer from similar symptoms?

>> **The degree of exposure:** Did your first noticeable asthma episode at work occur after a particularly significant exposure, such as a spill of chemicals or other industrial substances?

SEE YOUR DOCTOR

Depending on your condition's severity, your physician may prescribe medications that control your asthma symptoms at work. In most cases, however, for this treatment to be effective, your physician will probably advise you to find ways of avoiding or at least reducing your exposure to workplace triggers.

LATEX AND YOUR LUNGS

Although the incidence of latex allergy has been markedly reduced with the introduction of nonpowdered and nitrile gloves, latex is still occasionally used in medical facilities. It can be found in some medical gloves and medical equipment, such as latex ports in intravenous tubing for administration of fluids and medications. Your physician may test for serum specific IgE in order to distinguish latex causing an immediate IgE mediated reaction in contrast to the contact, delayed reaction which is a form of contact dermatitis caused by a type 4 delayed skin reaction.

Exposures can result in allergens from the rubber compounds sensitizing medical personnel. Latex is therefore considered a cause of occupational allergy and asthma in the healthcare industry. In addition, patients being treated in medical facilities may be exposed and sensitized to latex.

These exposures can lead to serious symptoms of allergic rhinitis, asthma, *urticaria* (hives), *angioedema* (deep swellings), and, in extreme cases, *anaphylaxis* (a potentially life-threatening reaction that affects many organs simultaneously).

(continued)

(continued)

The U.S. Food and Drug Administration (FDA) requires labeling of all medical devices and packaging containing natural rubber latex. Parents should be aware that latex-sensitive children can be at risk for severe respiratory reactions from inflating rubber balloons.

If you're at risk of developing allergic reactions to latex exposure, make sure that any healthcare professional who treats you knows this fact so you can, ideally, receive medical/dental care in a latex-free environment. This requires a setting in which no latex gloves are used, and no latex accessories (such as catheters, adhesives, tourniquets, and anesthesia equipment) come into contact with you. Similarly, if your occupation involves contact with latex, find out what you can do to avoid or minimize your exposure to this allergen. In healthcare settings, powder-free latex gloves and non-latex gloves and other latex-free medical equipment are increasingly available. Using these alternative products can substantially reduce the risk that you may suffer an allergic reaction to latex.

Additionally, wear a medical alert bracelet or pendant to alert medical personnel not to use latex products if you're unconscious or unable to communicate during a medical emergency. If you've experienced a serious allergic reaction to latex, also ask your physician whether an emergency epinephrine kit, such as an EpiPen, Auvi-Q, with an injectable dose of epinephrine, or nasally administered epinephrine (neffy) is advisable for you.

Avoiding Drug and Food Triggers

Some people with asthma also suffer from sensitivities to certain foods and medications which may potentially be life-threatening. In the following sections, we explain the most significant sensitivities that can adversely affect your asthma and what you can do to avoid them.

Aspirin sensitivities

Approximately 10 percent of asthma patients experience some level of sensitivity to aspirin, aspirin-containing compounds (such as Alka-Seltzer, Anacin, and Excedrin), and NSAIDs (Motrin, Advil, and Aleve). If your medical history includes nasal polyps and sinusitis in addition to asthma and aspirin sensitivity, use acetaminophen-based products such as Tylenol instead of aspirin or NSAIDs to relieve common aches and pains.

TECHNICAL STUFF

A more serious form of aspirin sensitivity is the *aspirin triad, also known as Aspirin Exacerbated Respiratory Disease (AERD).* This condition affects aspirin-intolerant patients who have asthma and chronic nasal polyps as well as a history of sinusitis. If you suffer from this form of aspirin sensitivity, adverse reactions to aspirin, aspirin-containing compounds, NSAIDs, and possibly newer prescription NSAIDs known as COX-2 inhibitors, including celecoxib (Celebrex), can result in severe or potentially life-threatening asthma attacks.

REMEMBER

We strongly advise anyone with this level of sensitivity to wear a MedicAlert bracelet or pendant. This device alerts medical personnel not to administer any medication to which you're sensitive if you're unconscious or unable to communicate during a medical emergency.

Beta-blockers

Physicians frequently prescribe oral beta-blocker medications, including Inderal, Lopressor, and Corgard, to treat conditions such as migraine headaches, high blood pressure, *angina* (chest pain), or *hyperthyroidism* (overactive thyroid), and beta-blocker eye drops for eye conditions such as glaucoma. If you have one of these disorders and you also have asthma, know that taking beta-blockers can worsen your asthma symptoms by blocking the beta$_2$-adrenergic receptor sites in your airways that cause *bronchodilation* (opening of the airways), thus making your asthma less responsive to beta$_2$-adrenergic (beta$_2$-agonist) bronchodilators.

WARNING

Occasionally, taking beta-blockers can trigger asthma episodes in susceptible individuals who haven't previously experienced any respiratory symptoms.

SEE YOUR DOCTOR

Because beta-blockers may trigger asthma symptoms, make sure that all physician you consult with for any of the conditions we mention in this section knows you have asthma and is informed of your complete medical history. If beta-blockers aren't advisable, your physician may prescribe alternative forms of medication therapy, such as other families of *antihypertensives* (blood pressure medicine) or other types of antimigraine drugs.

Food allergies

Some people with asthma develop hypersensitivities to certain foods. Although some foods have the potential to cause anaphylaxis, they don't appear to significantly increase the underlying airway inflammation that's characteristic of asthma in most patients.

SEE YOUR
DOCTOR

If your infant or young child has food allergies, they may tend to develop other allergy-related problems. In this case, your physician should evaluate your child for possible signs of asthma and other atopic (allergic) diseases, such as allergic rhinitis and *atopic dermatitis* (eczema).

SEE YOUR
DOCTOR

If you've experienced an episode of anaphylaxis, ask your physician whether an emergency epinephrine kit, such as an EpiPen or Auvi-Q, or nasal epinephrine (neffy) is advisable for you. Wear a medical alert bracelet or necklace in case you're unable to speak during a reaction. If you're hungering for details on food allergies, turn to Chapter 15.

Managing Other Medical Conditions and Asthma

In addition to the triggers we discuss in this chapter, certain activities, illnesses, and syndromes can induce your asthma symptoms or make them worse. Properly, managing these precipitating factors is as vital to effectively controlling your asthma as avoiding allergens and irritants.

Rhinitis and sinusitis

Poorly managing allergic and nonallergic forms of rhinitis can lead to *sinusitis*. This infection of the sinuses can aggravate your asthma symptoms, especially if it isn't responsive to repeated courses of antibiotic treatment. If so, sinus surgery may be necessary to treat sinusitis and reestablish control over asthma symptoms. Studies show that asthma patients who effectively manage their rhinitis and sinusitis can significantly improve their asthma symptoms.

Because your respiratory tract is essentially a continuum — think of it as the united airway — treating your nose and sinuses can help treat the underlying airway inflammation that characterizes asthma. In fact, when dealing with serious respiratory diseases such as asthma, physicians increasingly consider it vital to treat the whole patient — not just the patient's lungs. For more information on dealing with sinusitis and other rhinitis complications, turn to Chapter 7.

Gastroesophageal reflux disease (GERD)

The digestive disorder *gastroesophageal reflux disease* (GERD) occurs when the valve that separates the esophagus from the stomach doesn't function properly.

As a result, stomach acid and undigested food can wash up into the esophagus (and occasionally, through inhalation, into the respiratory tract) from the stomach in individuals who suffer from GERD. You can see a cross-section of the organs involved in GERD in Figure 9-2.

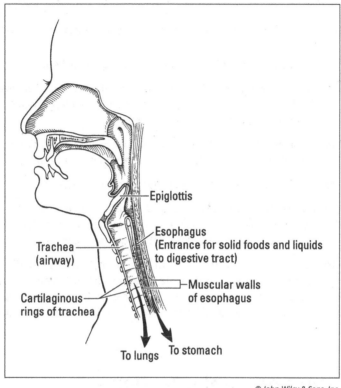

FIGURE 9-2: GERD occurs when stomach contents spill over into the esophagus.

© John Wiley & Sons, Inc.

Patients who suffer from GERD often burp during and after meals, complain of an acid taste in their mouth, and feel a burning sensation in their throat or chest, symptoms they typically describe as heartburn or indigestion.

GERD is a trigger of asthma symptoms in many patients with asthma and isa major trigger of adult-onset asthma (see Chapter 1) in patients whose asthma symptoms (coughing, wheezing, shortness of breath) aren't usually associated with allergic triggers. If you live with asthma, the flow of acidic digestive contents into your respiratory tract can make your underlying airway inflammation worse. GERD, with or without inhalation of stomach contents, has also been associated with increased bronchospasm and chronic cough due to irritation of the esophagus. Conversely, when asthma is active, it can aggravate GERD, and some of the drugs used to treat asthma, such as long-acting beta$_2$-adrenergic bronchodilators, can also worsen GERD symptoms.

If you have frequent heartburn and poorly controlled asthma, particularly with episodes that occur at night and disturb your sleep, you and your physician should consider the possibility that GERD contributes to your asthma symptoms.

To help ease the effects of GERD, your physician may advise the following:

>> Avoid eating or drinking within 3 hours of going to bed.

>> Avoid heavy meals and minimize dietary fat. Also, try to eat several small meals over the course of the day instead of fewer large meals, especially avoiding a large, heavy meal for dinner.

>> Eliminate or cut down on the consumption of aspirin, chocolate, peppermint, alcoholic beverages, coffee, tea, and carbonated beverages.

>> Avoid smoking and the use of any tobacco products.

>> Try elevating the head of your bed, by using 6- to 8-inch blocks, so that your stomach contents are less likely to rise to the point that you can inhale them while sleeping. Adding pillows under your head can also be of some benefit.

>> To control the digestive problems that result from your GERD symptoms, consider the use of appropriate OTC products, including Tagamet, Axid, and Pepcid AC. Your physician may also recommend medications such as Nexium, Protonix, Aciphex, and Prevacid, which decrease *gastric* (stomach) acid secretion.

Common viral infections

Viral respiratory infections, such as the common cold, flu, or COVID-19 and other coronavirus disease (see the next section for more information), can aggravate airway inflammation and trigger asthma symptoms. Children younger than 10 with asthma are particularly prone to asthma symptoms precipitated by *rhinovirus infections* (upper respiratory infections, usually referred to as the common cold).

Rhinovirus infections cause bronchial hyperreactivity and promote respiratory airway inflammation, leading to increased asthma symptoms. For infants and toddlers, viral infections of all types are the most common cause of severe asthma episodes because young children have smaller airways that are often more susceptible to bronchial obstruction. These infections are also the most common cause of episodes in adults, especially those with nonallergic (intrinsic) asthma.

WHAT TO DO ABOUT THE FLU

Antiviral medications can help you avoid coming down with influenza even when you've had a flu shot. Flu vaccines consist of the World Health Organization's (WHO) best guess of the viruses from the preceding year that may cause the flu during next year's influenza season. However, the WHO's predictions aren't always perfectly accurate. As a result, a flu shot may not fully protect you against the viral strains that cause the current year's flu epidemic, thus making antiviral medications extremely beneficial.

SEE YOUR DOCTOR

Inform your physician whenever you experience flu or cold symptoms. As comforting as you may find chicken soup when you're sniffly and sneezy, you may require early and aggressive medication therapy to keep the virus from adversely affecting your asthma.

Consider the following measures when you're dealing with viral infections:

>> If you have persistent asthma, ask your physician about receiving an annual flu vaccine to reduce the risk of suffering from an influenza respiratory infection that may aggravate your asthma symptoms.

REMEMBER

>> Prescription antiviral medications, such as zanamivir by inhalation (Relenza) and oseltamivir phosphate by oral tablet (Tamiflu), can stop the flu in its tracks and get you back on your feet sooner if you take them within the first two days of developing flu symptoms. Common flu symptoms include high fever, muscle aches, fatigue, and increased respiratory symptoms. Using these antiviral products can reduce the respiratory complications that accompany influenza infections, making these medications especially beneficial if you have asthma. However, antiviral medications are only for influenza and aren't effective against the common cold.

SEE YOUR DOCTOR

>> If your young child or infant experiences repeated viral infections that cause coughing and wheezing episodes, and your family medical history includes *atopy* (the genetic susceptibility for the immune system to produce antibodies to common allergens, which leads to allergy symptoms), make sure your physician evaluates your child for the possibility of asthma. (See Dr. Berger's book *Asthma For Dummies* [John Wiley & Sons, Inc.] for more information on childhood asthma.

COVID and asthma

You're probably familiar with the symptoms of coronavirus disease: high temperature, chills, a new continuous cough, changes to your normal sense of smell or taste, shortness of breath, fatigue, headache, sore throat, blocked nose, loss of appetite, and gastrointestinal upset. Some of these symptoms, such as breathlessness and coughing, are similar to asthma symptoms, but high temperature, tiredness, and change in taste or smell aren't characteristic of an asthma attack and are more likely due to a coronavirus infection.

SEE YOUR DOCTOR

If you test positive for COVID with these symptoms, you need to stay home and avoid contact with other people. Most people can manage their symptoms at home if they get lots of fluids and plenty of rest and maintain close fever control. Although studies have shown that most people with asthma aren't at higher risk from coronavirus, some patients with asthma may be more at risk from coronavirus if they're affected by the following factors:

>> Their asthma is uncontrolled.

>> They aren't taking their medications as prescribed.

>> They smoke.

>> They're overweight.

>> They have other health conditions, such as heart disease or diabetes.

TIP

The message is clear: Keep taking your asthma medicines as you normally would and follow your asthma action plan to keep yourself on track if COVID worsens your asthma symptoms. Contact your physician for guidance on any additional needed treatments, such as antivirals like nirmatrelvir and ritonavir (Paxlovid).

SEE YOUR DOCTOR

It can take a while to recover from coronavirus infections, even relatively mild ones. Be sure to continue treating your asthma as usual. Most people will get better within 4 weeks, but others may need 12 weeks or longer to recover. Symptoms that persist beyond 12 weeks may be due to long COVID, according to some experts. Some symptoms of long COVID, such as shortness of breath, persistent cough, chest pain, and fatigue, can resemble asthma symptoms. If you aren't getting better, consult your physician and consider asking for a referral to a specialist who can further evaluate and treat your condition.

Vaccinations as a preventative therapy

Because people with asthma are particularly vulnerable to complications and bad outcomes with viral respiratory infections, we strongly suggest these individuals get appropriate vaccinations. These include pneumonia, influenza, and COVID vaccinations. Adults, 60 years and over, should also be vaccinated against respiratory syncytial virus (RSV).

Contact your physician's office to arrange a schedule for these important preventative measures. Benjamin Franklin's famous comment that "*an ounce of prevention is worth a pound of cure*" is good advice even today.

Chapter **10**

Living Well with Asthma

Developing and sticking to a long-term asthma management strategy is a priceless investment in your overall health and quality of life, especially if you have persistent asthma. The fundamental guideline is to address the root cause of your symptoms: the underlying airway inflammation that characterizes asthma. In most cases, after patients realize how much better they feel when they effectively manage their asthma on a consistent basis, they don't go back to an ineffective short-term, crisis-management approach for dealing with their disease.

This chapter discusses how to proactively manage your asthma over the long term, which means developing a comprehensive asthma management plan to manage and monitor your condition. We will examine how to identify the four levels of asthma severity and outline the stepwise treatment approach, including the medications and various lung function tests that your physician may recommend to control your asthma and allow you to live a healthy and active life with asthma.

Outlining What a Long-Term Management Plan Includes

A comprehensive long-term management plan for asthma should include the following elements:

>> Undergoing objective testing and monitoring of your lung functions to initially diagnose your condition and to continuously assess the effectiveness of your treatment.

>> Avoiding and controlling exposure to asthma triggers and precipitating factors, such as other medical conditions (see Chapter 9).

>> Developing a safe and effective medication program that results in minimal or no adverse side effects and includes routinely taking appropriate long-term controller medications and using appropriate short-term quick-relief rescue medications if your symptoms suddenly get worse. For more information on asthma medications see Dr. Berger's book *Asthma For Dummies* (John Wiley & Sons, Inc.).

>> Initiating *pharmacotherapy* (treatment with medications) with a *stepwise* (step-up or step-down) approach (see the section "Following the Stepwise Approach" later in this chapter).

>> Consulting with an asthma specialist, such as an allergist or *pulmonologist* (lung physician), when advisable.

>> Tailoring your asthma management plan to your specific circumstances and condition, and continually educating yourself and your family about asthma and your specific condition (refer to the section "Understanding Self-Management" later in this chapter).

"OUTGROWING" YOUR ASTHMA: FACT OR FICTION?

Asthma isn't something you usually outgrow. Extensive studies have shown that asthma is an ongoing physical condition that doesn't just disappear forever when you feel better. Your asthma can vary in its symptoms and severity during your lifetime. However, just like the color of your eyes or your individual fingerprint pattern, when you have asthma, it remains another of your distinctive, although unseen, physical characteristics.

The airways of your lungs get bigger as you grow, so if you have asthma, mild airway obstruction may not affect you as much as you get older. Also, as you mature, your sensitivities may not be sufficient to cause noticeable clinical symptoms. However, people who feel that they "outgrew" their asthma as children or teenagers commonly experience symptoms of the disease later in life, particularly in response to certain triggers (see Chapter 9 for more on asthma triggers).

Focusing on the Four Levels of Asthma Severity

Experts from various fields of medicine have classified the severity of asthma — whether it's allergic or nonallergic — into four levels. These asthma severity levels provide the basis for the stepwise management of the disease.

REMEMBER

These levels of severity aren't permanent or static. Asthma is a condition that can change throughout your life. The primary goal of the stepwise approach that we describe in this chapter is to get the severity of your asthma to the lowest classification possible. Effectively treating your condition is crucial; otherwise, your asthma severity may move up the classification scale, deteriorating to the point where you may suffer from severe, relentless symptoms that adversely affect your quality of life.

As described in the National Institutes of Health (NIH) Guidelines for the Diagnosis and Management of Asthma, the four levels of asthma severity are

>> **Intermittent:** Symptoms occur no more than twice a week during the day and no more than twice a month at night. Lung-function testing shows 80 percent or greater of the predicted normal value, compared to reference values based on your age, height, sex, and race, as established by the American Thoracic Society. In addition, your peak expiratory flow rate (PEFR; see Chapter 3) doesn't vary by more than 20 percent during episodes and from morning to evening. Between episodes, you may be *asymptomatic* (not have noticeable symptoms), and your PEFR is normal. If your asthma is at this level, a worsening of symptoms is usually brief, lasting a few hours to a few days, with variations of intensity.

>> **Mild persistent:** Symptoms occur more than twice a week during the day, but less than once a day, and more than twice a month at night. Lung-function testing shows 80 percent or greater of the predicted normal value. Your PEFR may vary between 20 and 30 percent. If your asthma is at this level of severity, a worsening of symptoms can begin to affect your activities.

>> **Moderate persistent:** Symptoms occur daily and more than once a week at night, requiring daily use of a short-acting bronchodilator. Lung-function testing shows a 60 to 80 percent range of the normal predicted value. Your PEFR can vary more than 30 percent. Symptoms can worsen at least twice a week, with episodes lasting for days and affecting your activities.

>> **Severe persistent:** Symptoms occur continuously during the day and frequently at night, limiting physical activity. Lung-function testing is 60 percent or less of the normal predicted value. Your PEFR may vary more than 30 percent, and frequent aggravations of your condition can develop.

SEE YOUR DOCTOR

When diagnosing your condition, your physician should classify the severity of your asthma. Check to see which of the severity levels your condition most resembles, based on the definitions we list in this section. Your own symptoms and lung functions may not always fit neatly into one of these particular severity levels. Your physician should therefore evaluate your individual condition and develop a treatment plan for you based on the specific characteristics of your asthma. Keep in mind, however, that based on symptom criteria and the results of lung-function testing, most asthma patients have some form of persistent asthma — mild, moderate, or severe — requiring long-term control therapy.

SEE YOUR DOCTOR

If the symptoms you're experiencing seem to indicate that in fact, you have persistent asthma, the guidelines strongly advise having your lung functions evaluated by *spirometry* if you haven't already done so (see the section "Assessing Your Lungs" later in this chapter). To have a spirometry evaluation, you may need to ask your physician for a referral to an asthma specialist, such as an allergist or pulmonologist, because many primary care physicians don't have easy access to a spirometer.

Following the Stepwise Approach

Asthma severity levels are like steps in a staircase to controlling asthma, as shown in Figure 10-1. The basic concept of *stepwise management* is to initially prescribe long-term and quick-relief medications based on the severity level that's one step higher than the severity level you're experiencing (see Table 10-1). By using this approach, your physician can usually help you gain rapid control over your symptoms. After your condition has been under control for at least a month (in most cases), your physician can then reduce the level of your medications by one level (*step down*).

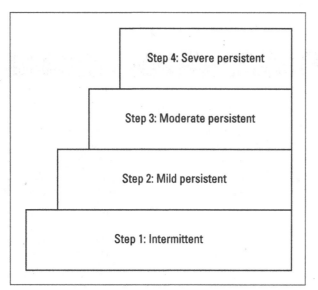

© John Wiley & Sons, Inc.

FIGURE 10-1: The steps of asthma severity levels.

REMEMBER

Using the stepwise approach to asthma management means that you *step up* your medication therapy to gain control, and then *step down* your medication therapy to maintain control. Regular monitoring of your PEFR and follow-up visits with your physician are vital to ensuring that you stay in step, as we explain in the next section.

The information in Table 10-1 is based on the NIH Guidelines for the Diagnosis and Management of Asthma. Remember that these are guidelines. Your physician should always evaluate your specific condition and prescribe individualized targeted therapy.

Stepping down

If you're on long-term maintenance medication at any level, your physician should review your treatment every one to six months. A gradual stepwise reduction in treatment may be possible after your symptoms are kept under good control, meaning that you feel well, have maintained improved lung function, and experienced no asthma symptoms.

REMEMBER

The goal of the stepwise approach is to use early and aggressive treatment to gain rapid control over your asthma symptoms, thus allowing your physician to reduce your medication to the lowest level required to maintain control of your condition.

TABLE 10-1   Stepwise Approach for Managing Asthma in Adults and Children Older Than 12

Step	Level	Preferred	Alternative
Step 1	Intermittent	PRN SABA	None
Step 2	Persistent	Daily low-dose ICS and PRN SABA	Daily LTRA and PRN SABA
Step 3*	Persistent	Daily and PRN combination low-dose ICS-formoterol	Daily medium-dose ICS and PRN SABA or daily low-dose ICS-LABA or daily low-dose ICS + LAMA
Step 4*	Persistent	Daily and PRN combination medium-dose ICS-formoterol	Daily medium-dose ICS-LABA or daily medium-dose ICS + LAMA and PRN SABA
Steps 2–4			Consider use of subcutaneous immunotherapy (allergy shots) as adjunct treatment to standard pharmacotherapy (medication)
Step 5	Persistent	Daily medium/high-dose ICS-LABA + LAMA and PRN SABA	Daily medium/high-dose ICS-LABA Consider adding asthma biologic (injection or infusion)
Step 6	Persistent	Daily high-dose ICS + LABA + oral systemic corticosteroids + PRN SABA	Consider adding asthma biologic (injection or infusion)

*If your asthma severity is at Step 3 or Step 4, consult an asthma specialist, such as an allergist or pulmonologist (lung physician), to achieve better control of your condition.

Abbreviations: ICS = inhaled corticosteroid; LABA = long-acting beta$_2$-agonist; LAMA = long-acting muscarinic antagonist; LTRA = leukotriene receptor antagonist; PRN = as necessary; SABA = inhaled short-acting beta$_2$-agonist.

Stepping up

SEE YOUR DOCTOR

If you find yourself frequently needing to use your quick-relief medications, your symptoms aren't under control, and your physician should consider increasing your treatment by one step. In assessing whether to step up your therapy, your physician will probably evaluate the following aspects of your current treatment step:

>> Your inhaler technique (refer to the section "Evaluating your inhaler technique" later in this chapter).

>> Your level of adherence in taking the medications your physician has prescribed.

REMEMBER

Take your prescriptions as your physician instructs is vital. If you're having trouble with a medication (because of potential side effects) or you don't understand the instructions, tell them so they can take appropriate measures.

>> Your exposure level to asthma triggers, such as allergens and irritants, and precipitating factors, such as viral infections and other medical conditions. Control your exposure to asthma triggers and precipitating factors as much as possible, no matter which step of treatment you're receiving (see Chapter 9 for information on controlling asthma triggers).

Make sure your asthma management plan clearly outlines at what point you should contact your physician if your symptoms are getting worse (refer to the section "Outlining What a Long-Term Management Plan Includes" earlier in this chapter).

Treating severe episodes in stepwise management

Your physician may consider prescribing a short rescue course of oral corticosteroids at any step if you suddenly experience a severe asthma episode and your respiratory condition abruptly deteriorates.

TIP

Discuss the risks of using oral corticosteroids with your physician. Recent studies have reported that more than four courses of this type of treatment in a lifetime may cause increased side effects like diabetes, heart disease, cataracts, and bone thinning.

WARNING

In some cases, severe episodes can occur even if your asthma is classified as intermittent. Many patients with intermittent asthma may experience severe and potentially life-threatening episodes, often because of upper respiratory viral infections (such as flu or colds), even though they otherwise have extended periods of normal or near-normal lung function and few clinically noticeable asthma symptoms.

Assessing Your Lungs

Objective measurements of your lung functions are essential for monitoring the severity of your asthma. You and your physician should regularly check your airways to determine whether you're at the right step of asthma medication. In addition to recording your asthma symptoms in a daily symptom diary (check out the section "Keeping symptom records" later in this chapter), you should obtain objective measurements of your lung functions with spirometry and peak-flow monitoring.

The following sections outline the types of lung function tests that your physician would likely perform when assessing the severity of your asthma and ways that you can monitor your condition yourself.

What your treating physician should do: Spirometry

A *spirometer* is a machine that your physician or asthma specialist, such as an allergist or pulmonologist, uses for measuring airflow from your large and small airways before and 15 minutes after you've inhaled a short-acting bronchodilator. The spirometer helps your asthma specialist diagnose whether you have asthma and also allows your physician to follow your asthma's clinical course of treatment.

For adults and children older than 4 or 5, spirometry currently provides the most accurate way of determining whether airway obstruction exists and whether it's reversible. For information on other types of lung-function tests your doctor may recommend, see Chapter 8. For more information on diagnosing asthma in children younger than 4, see Dr. Berger's book *Asthma For Dummies* (John Wiley & Sons, Inc.).

What you can do: Peak-flow monitoring

A *peak-flow meter* (see Figure 10-2) allows you to monitor your lung functions at home. The readings from this handy tool may be used in diagnosing asthma and its severity and can also help your physician prescribe medications and monitor your treatment's effectiveness. Peak-flow monitoring can also provide important early warning signs that an asthma episode is approaching.

TIP

Children older than 4 or 5 who have asthma generally can use this small handheld device to measure their own PEFR. If your kid constantly questions your judgment (children often challenge their parents about almost everything), using a peak-flow meter can help them understand when their condition may require them to limit their activities. If your child understands that the decreased PEFR is indicating that they should not go to soccer practice on that particular day because of worsening asthma symptoms and a PEFR reduction, you may have more success in helping them control their asthma.

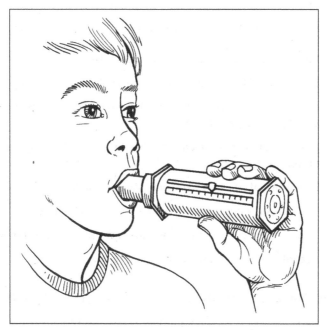

FIGURE 10-2:
A patient using a
peak-flow meter.

© John Wiley & Sons, Inc.

Explaining and using peak-flow meters for children

TIP

Parents may want to explain to their kids that when their peak-flow rate is down, it's like having an injury in their lungs. You can reinforce this analogy by telling your child that although the underlying airway inflammation isn't visible the problem still needs proper treatment, just as a sprained ankle needs to heal before they can resume normal activities.

By the same token, when your child's PEFR is between 80 and 100 percent of their personal best, you can breathe easier about encouraging sports and other physical activities that are a vital aspect of improving their overall health and fitness, including their lung functions. Make sure, however, that you and your child know how to manage potential symptoms of exercise-induced asthma (EIA), as explained in Chapter 9.

Using a peak-flow meter at home

TIP

Consider these basic instructions and tips for using most types of peak-flow meters (several different makes and models are currently available). Remember, however, to follow the instructions that come with your specific device. Ask your physician for advice on the most effective way you can use your peak-flow meter to assess your condition.

Generally, you use a peak-flow meter by following these steps:

1. **Move the sliding indicator at the base of the peak-flow meter to zero.**

2. **Stand up and take a deep breath to fully inflate your lungs.**

3. **Put the mouthpiece of the peak-flow meter into your mouth and close your lips tightly around it.**

4. **Blow as hard and as fast as possible, like you're blowing out the candles on your birthday cake.**

5. **Read the dial where the red indicator stopped.**

   The number opposite the indicator is your peak-flow rate.

6. **Reset the indicator to zero and repeat the process twice more.**

7. **Record the highest number that you reach.**

Finding your personal best peak-flow number

Your personal best peak-flow number is a measurement that reflects the highest number you can expect to achieve over a two- to three-week period after a course of aggressive treatment has produced good control of your asthma symptoms. Your best number is usually the result of step-up therapy.

TIP

To determine your personal best peak-flow number, take two peak-flow readings a day during an entire week when you're doing well and record the best result. Take one reading prior to taking medication in the morning and another reading between noon and 2 p.m. after using an inhaled short-acting bronchodilator. Compare your personal best peak-flow number with the measurement your physician predicts, which is based on national studies for children or adults of particular heights, sexes, and ages. This number can help you determine how your measurements compare with the national standards. When your asthma is well controlled, your PEFR should consistently read between 80 and 100 percent of your personal best.

WARNING

If your peak-flow measurements fall below 80 percent, prompt and aggressive intervention with medications and strict avoidance of potential asthma triggers may be necessary to prevent worsening symptoms. Ignoring a declining peak-flow reading can lead to serious symptoms and may result in the need for emergency treatment.

Reading green, yellow, and red peak-flow color zones

The peak-flow zone system involves green, yellow, and red areas that are similar to the lights on a traffic signal. Using your peak-flow meter on a regular basis enables you and your physician to treat symptoms before your condition deteriorates further.

TIP

You or your physician may want to place small pieces of colored tape next to the numbers on your peak-flow meter that correspond with the green, yellow, and red zones your physician provides as a graph on your written asthma peak-flow diary. (Refer to the section "Keeping symptom records" later in the chapter for more about asthma diaries.) Table 10-2 explains how to read the peak-flow color zones.

TABLE 10-2   **The Peak-Flow Color Zone System**

Zone	Meaning	Points to Consider
Green zone	Readings in this area are *safe*.	When your reading falls into the green zone, you've achieved 80 to 100 percent of your personal best peak flow. No asthma symptoms are present, and your treatment plan is controlling your asthma. If your readings consistently remain in the green zone, you and your physician may consider reducing your daily medications.
Yellow zone	Readings in this area indicate *caution*.	When your readings fall into the yellow zone, you're achieving only 50 to 80 percent of your personal best peak flow. An asthma attack may be present, and your symptoms may worsen. You may need to step up your medication temporarily.
Red zone	Readings in this area mean *medical alert*.	Readings in the red zone mean that you've fallen below 50 percent of your personal best peak flow. These readings often signal the start of a moderate to severe asthma attack.

SEE YOUR DOCTOR

If your readings are often in the yellow zone, even after you take the appropriate quick-relief medication your asthma management plan specifies, contact your physician. If your readings are in the red zone, use your quick-relief bronchodilator and anti-inflammatory medications immediately (based on your individualized asthma management plan) and contact your physician if your PEFR doesn't immediately return to and remain in the yellow or green zone.

Taking Stock of Your Condition

In addition to obtaining an objective measurement of your lung function with measuring devices, keeping track of a variety of other indicators is an important aspect of controlling your asthma. Your most valuable tracking device is usually a daily symptom diary. In fact, you may want to develop a rating system (in a shared decision-making approach with your physician) for your diary that assesses your symptoms on a scale of 0 to 3, ranging from no symptoms to severe symptoms. Here we spell out what you need to know about recording your symptoms and keeping track of your meds.

Keeping symptom records

REMEMBER

You should monitor and record the following indicators in your daily symptom diary:

>> Your signs and symptoms, as well as their severity

>> Any coughing you experience

>> Any incidence of wheezing

>> Nasal congestion

>> Disturbances in your sleep, such as coughing or wheezing that awakens you

>> Any symptoms that affect your ability to function normally or reduce your normal activities

>> Anytime you miss school or work because of symptoms

>> How often you use your short-acting beta$_2$-adrenergic bronchodilator (rescue medication)

Tracking serious symptoms

REMEMBER

Your daily symptom diary is also the place to monitor symptoms that are severe enough to make you seek unscheduled office visits, after-hours treatments, emergency room visits, and hospitalizations. Therefore, you also want to note the date and type of treatment you have.

Be sure to record the following types of serious symptoms:

>> Breathlessness or panting while you're at rest

>> The need to remain in an upright position in order to breathe

>> Difficulty speaking

>> Agitation or confusion

>> An increased breathing rate of more than 30 breaths per minute

>> Loud wheezing while inhaling and/or exhaling

>> An elevated pulse rate of more than 120 heartbeats per minute

TIP

Furthermore, record any exposures to triggers or precipitating factors that may have caused asthma flare-ups, including

>> Irritants, such as chemicals and cigarette or fireplace smoke

>> Allergens, such as plant pollen, household dust, molds, and animal fur

>> Air pollution

>> Exercise (Chapter 9 provides more information on EIA)

>> Sudden changes in the weather, particularly cold temperatures and chilly winds

>> Reactions to beta-blockers (such as Inderal or Timoptic), aspirin, and related products, including nonsteroidal anti-inflammatory drugs (NSAIDs) and food additives (see Chapter 9)

>> Other medical conditions, such as upper respiratory viral infections (colds and flu), gastroesophageal reflux disease (GERD), and sinusitis (see Chapter 9)

Monitoring your medication use

REMEMBER

Recording all the side effects that you experience when taking your prescribed medication is also important. Various asthma medications include different levels of side effects that a person may experience. However, in most cases, patients who understand their asthma management plan and take their medications according to instructions have few, if any, adverse side effects.

Knowing and remembering the names of your medications is important, especially if you're taking multiple prescriptions for several conditions. The best approach is to keep an updated list of all your drugs in your smart device to review with your physician, especially if you're taking multiple medications. Unfortunately, telling your physician that you're on a "white inhaler" or "yellow pill" doesn't provide helpful information for preventing drug interactions with other medications.

Evaluating your inhaler technique

Your healthcare team should show you the correct way to use your inhaler and have you demonstrate your inhaler technique at each office visit. More than 70 percent of patients don't use their inhalers correctly, reduces its performance and effectiveness. It's vitally important to use your inhaler correctly with a valved holding chamber to direct the medication deep into your lungs where it's needed. Improper inhaler use is often the reason some patients have difficulty controlling their asthma symptoms.

Understanding Self-Management

It takes two (at least) to treat asthma. You and your physician (as well as your other healthcare providers) are partners in controlling your asthma. Other members of your asthma partnership can include nurses, pharmacists, and any healthcare professionals who treat you or assist you in understanding and effectively managing your condition.

Although asthma isn't contagious, if you have asthma, your family also has the condition because you all may need to deal with the various issues associated with your medical condition's treatment. In fact, studies show that family support can be a major positive influence in the success of any asthma treatment plan. Particularly important to your asthma treatment is making sure the people you live with (as well as coworkers, fellow students, or anyone you're around much of the time) help you reduce your exposure to asthma triggers and precipitating factors.

If your child has asthma, you should also be a partner with your child's physician and other medical professionals in their management of the condition.

Working with your physician

Participate in shared decision-making by developing treatment goals *with* your physician. Make sure that you understand how your asthma management plan (refer to the section "Outlining What a Long-Term Management Plan Includes" earlier in this chapter) works and that you can openly communicate with your physician and share your experience about the effects and results of your treatment.

Making sure your plan is tailored to your specific needs, as well as your family's, is also very important. This can include considering any cultural beliefs and practices that may have an impact on your perception of asthma and medication therapy. Openly discuss any such issues with your physician, so that together, you can develop an approach to asthma management that empowers you to take control of your condition. Ensuring that your plan is tailored to fit you and your family makes you a more motivated patient, which almost always means you'll be healthier.

Evaluating your plan for the long term

Successfully managing your asthma also means constantly evaluating your asthma management plan to determine whether it provides you with the means to achieve your asthma management goals.

REMEMBER

Always keep in mind that asthma is a variable, complex, multifaceted condition. Just as many other aspects of your life can change and vary over time, your asthma may also manifest in different ways throughout your life. Remember: Your goal is lifetime management of your condition.

Becoming an expert on your asthma

SEE YOUR DOCTOR

Your education about asthma and its treatment should begin as soon as you're diagnosed. Your physician should make sure you have a thorough understanding of all aspects of your condition. Your education should include factors such as the following:

>> Knowing the basic facts about asthma.

>> Understanding your asthma severity level, how it affects you, and advisable treatment methods.

>> Becoming familiar with all the elements of asthma self-management, including your specific condition, proper use of various inhalers and nebulizers, self-monitoring skills, and effective ways of avoiding triggers and allergy-proofing your home.

>> Developing a written individualized daily and emergency self-management plan with your input (see the section "Outlining What a Long-Term Management Plan Includes" earlier in this chapter).

>> Determining the level of support you receive from family and friends in treating your asthma. It's also important for your physician to help you identify an asthma partner from among your family members, relatives, or friends. This person should find out how asthma affects you and should understand your asthma management plan so they can assist (if necessary) if your condition suddenly worsens. It may help to include them in your physician visits.

>> Asking your physician or other members of your asthma management team for guidance in setting priorities when implementing your asthma

management plan. If you need to make environmental changes in your life, such as allergy-proofing your home (which may include relocating a pet, pulling up the carpets, installing air filtration devices, and many other steps explained in Chapter 5), you may want advice on which steps you need to take promptly and which steps can wait.

Improving Your Quality of Life

Taking asthma medication doesn't mean you can afford to ignore other aspects of your health. Managing your asthma for the long term also requires being healthy overall. The better you take care of yourself, the more success you'll have in treating your asthma and living a full, normal life.

REMEMBER

Consider these important commonsense guidelines as you develop an asthma management plan:

>> **Eat right.** A healthy, well-balanced diet is especially important for people who have asthma. Eat fresh fruits, lean meats, fish, grains, and a plentiful supply of vegetables.

>> **Sleep well.** If you experience asthma symptoms during the night that disturb your sleep, tell your physician. These types of symptoms should be treated, and they may indicate that you're susceptible to precipitating factors such as GERD or asthma triggers (see Chapter 9).

SEE YOUR DOCTOR

>> **Stay fit.** When patients are in good physical condition, their asthma is often easier to control. You don't have to sit on life's sidelines just because you have asthma. Your physician can prescribe medications that you can take preventively to control symptoms of EIA, thus enabling you to enjoy many types of exercise and sports activities in spite of your asthma. (Chapter 9 provides information on ways to control EIA.)

>> **Reduce stress.** By effectively controlling your asthma, you'll feel less anxious about your condition, thus reducing your overall levels of anxiety and further helping you manage your asthma.

With effective, appropriate care from your physician and your own motivated participation as a patient, your asthma management plan can enable you to lead a full and active life. However, if properly following your asthma management plan still doesn't allow you to participate fully in the activities and pursuits that matter to you, openly communicate this to your physician so you both can work together to adjust your plan and maximize the effectiveness of your treatment.

4

Understanding Allergic Skin Conditions

Diagnose your disorder so you can get the best medical help.

Know how to treat atopic dermatitis and find relief of your symptoms.

Classify the types of contact dermatitis so you can avoid substances that trigger your symptoms.

Understand the difference between urticaria and angioedema so you can treat each condition properly.

Distinguish allergic from nonallergic mechanisms and how they might be affecting your condition.

Chapter **11**

Controlling Atopic Dermatitis

Atopic dermatitis is more than just dry, itchy skin. It can affect your quality of life — especially in the case of children who suffer from this condition — and can lead to complications such as bacterial and viral skin infections.

REMEMBER

Atopic dermatitis (in Greek, *derma* is skin, and *itis* means inflammation), also known as *atopic eczema* (in Greek, *eczema* means to erupt or boil out) or *allergic eczema* (*atopy* refers to the genetic predisposition to develop allergies; see Chapter 1) frequently occurs in conjunction with allergic respiratory diseases, such as allergic rhinitis (commonly referred to as *hay fever*, as we explain in Chapter 4) and can also precede other allergic symptoms. Therefore, finding out that you have atopic dermatitis can provide the first clue that you're at higher risk of developing other allergies and asthma.

Key points to keep in mind about atopic dermatitis include the following:

>> An estimated 16.5 million adults in the United States suffer from atopic dermatitis, and more than half of those individuals already have or will develop asthma or allergic rhinitis.

>> More than 90 percent of patients with chronic atopic dermatitis are infected with the bacteria *Staphylococcus aureus* (a bacterial staph infection that causes *impetigo*, a contagious bacterial skin infection), which affects only 5 percent of people who don't have atopic dermatitis.

>> Approximately 10 percent of infants and children in the United States suffer from this skin problem, which can begin as early as two months of age. Atopic dermatitis symptoms often become less severe as you mature, with reduced itching and scratching and lesions that aren't as severe. According to current research, up to 80 percent of children will outgrow atopic dermatitis; however, if you're diagnosed with severe disease at a young age and live in an urban area, your condition is more likely to persist into adulthood.

>> In children who have undergone double-blind, placebo-controlled oral food challenges (see Chapter 14), milk, egg, peanut, soy, wheat, and fish accounted for close to 90 percent of the food allergens found to worsen their symptoms of atopic dermatitis. In many of these cases, if parents make sure that their children's food allergies are identified — and the children avoid the implicated food — symptoms of atopic dermatitis and other allergies can be greatly reduced and, in some instances, may potentially stop altogether.

The Itch That Scratches or the Scratch That Itches

Although the heading of this section may seem like a "chicken or egg" question, the hallmark of atopic dermatitis is what physicians call the *itch-scratch cycle*. A related characteristic of atopic dermatitis is a lowered itch threshold, which means that an individual is much more prone to feeling itchy. The following sections take a deep-dive into atopic dermatitis, explaining its key characteristics, identifying its common names, and understanding how it appears in infants and children.

Examining this never-ending itching

These key aspects of the disease can initiate a vicious cycle of incessant itching: The inflammation caused by atopic dermatitis dries out the skin, producing an itchy feeling. This itchiness leads a person to scratch the itch, resulting in more irritation and inflammation, which further dries out the skin, making it even itchier, resulting in more scratching and increasingly damaged skin. Eventually, the skin is weakened to the point where fissures and cracks develop, allowing irritants, allergens, bacteria, and viruses to enter, triggering allergic reactions, or causing infections.

Other defining characteristics of atopic dermatitis include

>> Chronic or chronically relapsing *lesions* (irritated reddening) of the skin. On adults, these lesions commonly result in scarred, thickened skin with creased, accented lines, particularly in areas such as the palms and inside the elbows. These areas can develop a leathery texture.

With infants and children, these lesions may also affect the face, extremities, the creases of knees and elbow, and the trunk and neck areas, but not the diaper area (see Figure 11-1).

>> Chronic hand eczema may be the most common symptom of atopic dermatitis in many adult cases, but eczema can also affect the neck, feet, and creases of the knees and elbows.

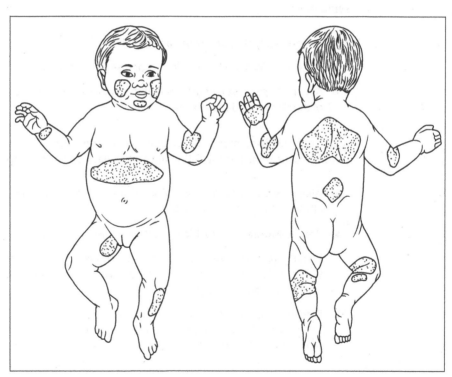

FIGURE 11-1: Eczema can affect many areas of a child's skin.

© *John Wiley & Sons, Inc.*

>> A personal or family history of asthma, allergic rhinitis, allergic rhinoconjuncti-vitis, food allergies, and atopic dermatitis often is associated with atopic dermatitis. However, in many cases involving infants or young children, evidence of other allergies may not be as obvious. When diagnosing atopic dermatitis in younger children, physicians may also look for minor signs, such as

- *Xerosis* (dry skin)

- *Ichthyosis* (white, dry and scaly skin)

- Severely lined palms

- Susceptibility to skin infections, especially herpes simplex (a virus that often causes fever blisters) and *Staphylococcus aureus*

- Dry skin around nipples

If your physician suspects that you suffer from atopic dermatitis, your physical examination also includes an evaluation of the following potential signs and symptoms:

>> Red and scaly skin, abrasions, and pimples

>> The extent, location (on your body), and severity of skin lesions

>> Any crusting or oozing pustules that may indicate infection, scaling, or scarring of the skin around the lesions

Also, your physician may look for evidence of atopy (allergic conditions) by deter-mining the presence of the following additional signs and symptoms:

>> **Allergic shiners:** Dark circles under your eyes that can provide evidence of allergic rhinitis (see Chapter 4).

>> **Dennie-Morgan infraorbital fold:** A small skin fold under the eyes.

>> **Recurrent conjunctivitis:** Redness over the eyeballs and on the underside of your eyelids, as well as swollen, itchy, and watery eyes (see Chapter 6 for more information on this allergy).

>> **Side effects:** Such as furrowed or thin, shiny skin, a result of chronic overuse of topical corticosteroid medications (we explain the appropriate uses of these medications in "Taking medications" later in this chapter).

Naming your disorder

Most patients (and even some physicians) often use the terms *eczema* and *atopic dermatitis* interchangeably. However, in medical terms, *eczema* refers more generally to a severe inflammatory itchy skin condition (sometimes also described as the "itch that rashes") that is one of the most common symptoms of atopic dermatitis as well as other conditions, including:

>> Skin inflammations, such as seborrheic dermatitis, irritant dermatitis, and contact dermatitis (see Chapter 12). In particular, physicians often need to evaluate patients over 16 with eczema symptoms for contact dermatitis.

>> Scabies, herpes simplex infections, recurrent *Staphylococcus aureus*, and HIV.

>> Psoriasis and other nonallergic, noninfectious chronic inflammatory skin conditions.

If you have eczema, your physician may advise you to undergo certain medical tests to determine whether the underlying cause of your skin inflammation has an allergic basis or is instead the result of an infectious organism. They may also supplement these tests by taking small samples of a lesion for culture and identification of suspected bacterial, viral, or fungal agents.

Most people with eczema have unusually high levels of total IgE antibodies and eosinophils (see Chapter 2). Therefore, your physician may further recommend allergy skin testing and/or specific Immunocap blood testing (see Chapter 3) to identify any particular allergens that may be triggering your skin symptoms.

Identifying infant issues

REMEMBER

Atopic dermatitis rarely occurs in infants under 6 weeks of age. If a baby has an eczema rash in the first month of life, your physician needs to evaluate the infant for the possibility of an immunodeficiency disorder. In the vast majority of cases, they aren't evaluating your baby specifically for AIDS (just one out of a whole multitude of immune deficiency diseases) but instead, they're attempting to rule out other types of diseases (see Chapter 2).

Other special considerations for infants with skin conditions include

>> **Diaper dermatitis:** This type of skin rash isn't a typical allergic reaction. A skin infection or contact dermatitis is a more probable cause of diaper rash.

>> **Seborrheic dermatitis:** With babies, distinguishing seborrheic dermatitis from atopic dermatitis may prove difficult. If your infant's armpit, diaper area, and top of head (cradle cap) show signs of eczema, seborrheic dermatitis is the more likely cause.

Exploring atopic dermatitis in children

The earlier the onset of atopic dermatitis, the more severe the problem. Because 60 percent of patients with atopic dermatitis develop signs of this disease before their first birthday, this condition is especially problematic for parents caring for affected infants and young children.

Youngsters with atopic dermatitis often infect their skin by scratching themselves with fingers that are full of all sorts of bacteria. As any parent knows, kids can get really dirty very fast. Keeping infants and young children from scratching their itchy skin is one of the main challenges in treating and managing atopic dermatitis — they just don't understand why they shouldn't scratch. Refer to the section "Treating Atopic Dermatitis" later in the chapter where we provide tips on how to break, or at least control, the itch–scratch cycle — the key to managing atopic dermatitis.

WARNING

Infants and children who show signs of atopic dermatitis (such as eczema) are often at a greater risk of subsequently developing other allergies. If your child has eczema and other signs of atopic dermatitis, watch out for other types of symptoms, such as coughing, a scratchy throat, or runny nose. Instead of indicating a cold, these symptoms may serve as early warning signs of allergic rhinitis and/or asthma.

DOCTOR SAYS

A TRUE STORY FROM DR. BERGER

As a child, I suffered from atopic dermatitis, so I can truly relate to the children with this type of allergy. Atopic dermatitis is a miserable condition and is an especially serious and traumatic problem for children. I remember scratching incessantly at night. Wearing shorts and short-sleeve shirts was embarrassing because I didn't want people to see the bleeding behind my knees and elbows. Fortunately, my condition improved with age. However, I still have occasional flare-ups, mostly on my hands and fingers, because my profession as a physician has required me to repeatedly wash my hands, which leads to a constant drying effect on my skin.

Treating Atopic Dermatitis

Successful management of atopic dermatitis requires a systematic, multi-pronged approach based on these key steps (which the following discusses):

» Moisturizing and softening your skin to keep it from drying out.

» Identifying and eliminating (as much as possible) irritants, allergens, sources of infection, and causes of emotional stress.

» Using topical corticosteroid preparations, such as hydrocortisone (Hytone), triamcinolone (Kenalog), mometasone (Elocon), and fluticasone (Cutivate) to control the inflammatory symptoms of allergic reactions. Your physician may also prescribe other medications, depending on your condition.

REMEMBER

The only way to manage atopic dermatitis is to control the itching. To illustrate this point, physicians often ask parents of children with atopic dermatitis to compare the appearance of their children's arms and legs with their backs. Although your children's limbs may appear extremely scratched and inflamed, their backs usually look far better. (Kids have a hard time reaching around to scratch their backs — if they can't scratch it, they won't damage it.) Therefore, keeping your children's fingernails short, instituting effective topical measures (such as using emollient soaps and moisturizers), and administering prescribed topical and/or oral medications are all essential to help control itching and keep the scratching damage to a minimum.

Moisturizing your skin

The first line of defense against atopic dermatitis is maintaining moist skin. In many cases, making sure your skin doesn't dry out provides dramatic relief of your symptoms. We suggest developing a regular routine of skin care that includes taking baths with products that help your skin absorb moisture and applying creams, lotions, and ointments immediately after bathing to lubricate and moisturize your skin. An effective skin moisturizing routine may also reduce your need for topical corticosteroid medications.

TIP

One of the simplest and most effective ways to relieve symptoms of atopic dermatitis is to take lukewarm soaking baths for 20 to 30 minutes. Avoid hot baths or showers because the heat increases itching and skin dryness.

Keep these other points in mind when bathing:

>> Adding oatmeal (Aveeno) or baking soda to your bath water may provide a soothing effect, but doing so won't help moisturize your skin.

>> Use a mild bar soap (Dove, Basis) or a non-soap cleanser with neutral pH (Cetaphil). Avoid using bubble bath or bath oils because they can form a barrier that prevents the bath water from moisturizing your skin. If you find oil especially soothing, add it to your bath after you get in the water to seal in the moisture.

>> Dry yourself gently by patting your skin with a soft towel; avoid rubbing briskly.

>> Apply emollient cream (CeraVe, Eucerin, Aquaphor) or lotion (CeraVe, Keri) to retain your skin's moisture within three minutes after drying off. Even Crisco shortening has been used effectively as an inexpensive moisturizer. *Tip:* Creams, which are thicker in consistency than lotions, are useful during the drier winter season.

We strongly advise against using lotions with high water or alcohol content because these products usually evaporate quickly, leaving your skin dry. Likewise, avoid lotions and creams that contain preservatives, solubilizers, fragrances, and astringents because these ingredients can dry and irritate your skin. Check the label to see whether the product contains these ingredients.

Avoiding triggers of atopic dermatitis

As with other allergic conditions, avoidance is a vital aspect of effectively managing atopic dermatitis. Although you may not be able to eliminate or avoid all allergy triggers and irritants in your environment, taking reasonable steps to identify, eliminate, and avoid factors that worsen or aggravate your atopic dermatitis can often provide enough relief to substantially improve your quality of life.

Irritants

In addition to the common irritants of asthma, allergic rhinitis, and sinusitis which we list in Chapter 5, you also should try to avoid materials, substances, and conditions that can trigger the scratch–itch cycle. Materials and situations to avoid include

>> **Abrasive clothing:** We usually advise patients to wear open-weave, loose-fitting cotton, or cotton-blended clothes. We also suggest laundering new clothes before wearing them to get as many of the chemicals, especially formaldehyde, out of the fabric as possible.

>> **Detergent:** Avoid residual detergent in laundered clothes. Try using liquid detergent and adding a second rinse cycle to remove more detergent during washing.

>> **Temperature extremes:** In winter, an area humidifier can help keep your skin from drying out and cracking, especially if your home has central heating. In the summer, use air conditioning to maintain a comfortable climate indoors and to remove excess humidity.

>> **Sports:** Avoid conditions or activities that involve heavy perspiration, intense physical contact, or heavy clothing. However, children with atopic dermatitis needs to remain as normally active as possible. Swimming may serve as an acceptable activity, although children should learn to rinse the chlorine off as soon as they get out of the pool and to apply moisturizer to their skin immediately after drying.

TIP

Sunlight can benefit people with atopic dermatitis as long as you don't get a sunburn, overheat, or perspire excessively. However, make sure that you use sunscreen when you expose yourself to the sun. Because sunscreens can irritate your skin, find one that doesn't trigger your atopic dermatitis symptoms.

Allergens

Inhalant allergens such as pollens, molds, dust, and animal dander, which are common triggers of allergic rhinitis, can sometimes trigger symptoms of atopic dermatitis. (We provide an extensive survey of these allergens in Chapter 5.) Key points to keep in mind about inhalant allergens and atopic dermatitis include the following:

>> Some patients experience atopic dermatitis symptoms that worsen with seasonal changes, which inhalant allergens, such as ragweed pollen, may cause.

>> Exposure to dander (especially from household pets), dust mites, and molds may cause perennial atopic dermatitis symptoms. If your symptoms worsen (especially around your face and head) during the night while you sleep, dust mites (see Chapter 4) may be the problem. Consider taking steps to allergy-proof your home, or at least your bedroom against these microscopic creatures. (See Chapter 5 for avoidance and allergy-proofing steps, as well as more dust mite details.)

Infections

Skin infections and complications can recur regularly with atopic dermatitis. Common infectious agents include herpes simplex (viral), *Staphylococcus aureus* (bacterial), scabies (mite infestation), and *dermatophyte* (fungal) infections.

The keys to avoiding these infections involve breaking the itch-scratch cycle and maintaining well-moisturized skin. Refer to the section "Moisturizing your skin" earlier in this chapter.

Stress

We all have times when we let upsetting events and pressures get to us. However, if you have atopic dermatitis, feelings of frustration, embarrassment, anger, and hostility may lead you to scratch more, thus worsening your skin's condition.

TIP

Professional counseling can help you if your state of mind adversely affects your ability to manage atopic dermatitis.

Taking medications

SEE YOUR DOCTOR

If your symptoms don't improve as a result of the self-care and avoidance measures that we describe earlier in this chapter, or if your eczema is severe, your physician may prescribe specific medications to treat your condition (we cover several here).

Topical corticosteroids

Topical corticosteroid medications, applied directly to the affected skin area, are a mainstay of eczema treatment because of their anti-inflammatory action. Physicians currently use seven classes of topical corticosteroids (Ranked according to strength, as we explain in Table 11-1) to treat symptoms of atopic dermatitis. These products are available in cream, ointment, and lotion forms. You should keep the following in mind the using topical corticosteroids to treat atopic dermatitis:

>> Your physician should instruct you on the proper and safe application of topical corticosteroids. In general, avoid using high-potency preparations on your face, eyelids, armpits, or genital areas. For those areas, use low-potency topical corticosteroids.

>> Your physician should prescribe high-potency topical corticosteroids only for a short time and only for use on scarred and thickened skin areas. A two-to three-week course of low-potency medication generally follows your high-potency prescription.

>> Use topical corticosteroids with emollients to help keep your skin moisturized.

>> The lowest potency topical corticosteroid at the lowest dosage that will control your atopic dermatitis symptoms is the preparation that you should use, based on your physician's recommendation.

TABLE 11-1

Topical Corticosteroid Classes Ranked from Highest Potency (Group 1) to Lowest Potency (Group 7)

Potency	Active Ingredient	Formulation	Brand Name
Group 1	Clobetasol	0.05% ointment/cream	Temovate
	Betamethasone	0.05% ointment/cream	Diprolene
Group 2	Mometasone	0.1% ointment	Elocon
	Halcinonide	0.1% cream	Halog
	Fluocinonide	0.05% ointment/cream	Lidex
	Desoximetasone	0.25% ointment/cream	Topicort
Group 3	Fluticasone	0.005% ointment	Cutivate
	Halcinonide	0.1% ointment	Halog
	Betamethasone	0.1% ointment	Valisone
Group 4	Mometasone	0.1% cream	Elocon
	Triamcinolone	0.1% ointment/cream	Kenalog
	Fluocinolone	0.025% ointment	Synalar
Group 5	Fluocinolone	0.025% cream	Synalar
	Hydrocortisone	0.2% ointment	Westcort
Group 6	Desonide	0.05% ointment/cream/lotion	DesOwen
	Alclometasone	0.05% ointment/cream	Aclovate
Group 7	Hydrocortisone	2.5% and 1% ointment/cream	Hytone

WARNING

Before using topical corticosteroids with children, make sure that your physician explains the potential adverse side effects. In some cases, highly potent topical corticosteroids may be absorbed through the skin into the blood circulation. This can potentially suppress the function of adrenal glands, particularly in children (due to their thinner skin), resulting in rare cases, in a reduced rate of growth. Local side effects, at the site of application can include skin *atrophy* (thinning), stretch marks, and infections. The base used in some types of topical corticosteroid creams and ointments can also cause skin irritations. Notify your physician immediately if any of these side effects occur.

Antibiotics

In cases where bacterial skin infections occur, your physician may prescribe a short course of an anti-staphylococcal antibiotic such as cephalosporin or erythromycin. You may apply some of the antibiotics, such as mupirocin (Bactroban), used to treat local bacterial skin infections, directly to the affected area as topical preparations, but oral antibiotics are generally more effective and have less potential for causing skin irritation than topical antibiotic preparations.

If your skin infections don't respond to antibiotics, herpes or some other type of viral infection may be the underlying cause. In such cases, your physician may refer to you to a dermatologist to diagnose your condition.

Antihistamines

Oral antihistamines, according to the most recent guidelines, aren't routinely recommended for the itching associated with atopic dermatitis. The evidence for reduction of *pruritis* (itching) in eczema isn't clear. Research has found that eczema activates cells that involve a different set of nerve cells compared to the cells that carry itch signals, which would normally respond to antihistamines.

REMEMBER

However, if patients can't sleep because of the severity of their atopic dermatitis symptoms (for example, intense itching), physicians may take advantage of the drowsy side effects of OTC antihistamines by prescribing an a.m./p.m. dosing regimen:

>> **At night:** A sedating antihistamine. Taking an OTC antihistamine such as Benadryl in the evening may help patients relax and sleep (the active ingredient in Benadryl is the same ingredient as in many sleep preparations), thus breaking the itch-scratch cycle (at least at night).

>> **During the day:** A nonsedating one (see Chapter 6 for more information on allergy medication). During the day, physicians may prescribe a nonsedating antihistamine, such as Allegra or Claritin, or a less sedating one, such as Zyrtec, to keep allergic reactions under control while still enabling patients to remain active and alert. However, physicians usually caution patients in these cases that the sedative side effects of the first-generation OTC antihistamine may still persist during the day.

Coal tar

Back in the old days, (even before Dr. Berger's time), coal tar preparations made from crude coal tar extracts were a mainstay of atopic dermatitis treatment. Although physicians don't use these older preparations much anymore (especially since the development of topical corticosteroids), you can find newer less-odorous coal tar products that effectively control itching and skin inflammation. In fact, some patients prefer to use coal tar medications as compounds in ointments or creams, such as 5 percent LCD (Liquor Carbonis Detergens), often reducing the need for more potent topical corticosteroid preparations. For example, in cases of scalp eczema, some physicians recommend tar shampoos (T/Gel, Ionil-T) as an effective treatment.

WARNING

Don't apply tar preparations on newly inflamed skin, your face, or other areas exposed to sunlight. Doing so can cause further inflammation and occasional photosensitivity reactions. Although the new coal tar preparations don't stain as much as the older products, be careful when using them near clothing, especially white or light-colored garments. Some physicians recommend that you use the preparation at bedtime and then wash it off in the morning, so you don't have to worry about odor or staining during the day.

Dealing with special cases

Your atopic dermatitis condition may require other, more specialized forms of treatment than the ones we describe in the chapter. Your physician may prescribe some of the following treatments for difficult-to-manage atopic dermatitis:

>> **Wet dressings:** These dressings can help prevent you from scratching and may also help absorb the topical corticosteroids through the outer layer of your skin. However, overusing wet dressings may result in dry and cracked skin unless you apply a moisturizer. Occasionally, your physician may advise using an occlusive (barrier) dressing such as plastic wrap, for short periods of time, to prevent evaporation of the preparation. Only apply these medications with dressings under your physician's supervision, and only use this type of treatment if you suffer from severe and chronic types of atopic dermatitis.

>> **Oral corticosteroids:** If you suffer from severe atopic dermatitis, and all other treatment options have been exhausted, you may rarely require a short course of oral corticosteroids. However, you may need to taper off the dosage of oral corticosteroids rather than stopping it abruptly, in order to avoid a syndrome called *rebound flaring*, in which your atopic dermatitis symptoms may suddenly reappear.

>> **Bleach baths:** Dilute bleach baths may be beneficial in patients with moderate and severe atopic dermatitis by killing bacteria on the skin and reducing itching, redness, and scaling. This is usually prepared by adding a half cup of household bleach to a full tub of water, soaking for about 10 minutes, and then rinsing off. This treatment is usually recommended two to three times per week.

>> **Phototherapy:** This treatment, which uses ultraviolet (UV) light, can effectively treat some cases of chronic atopic dermatitis. However, only consider phototherapy if it's administered under the supervision of a dermatologist.

>> **Photochemotherapy:** A recently developed treatment that combines UV light and the drug methoxysporalen is known as *photochemotherapy*. Due to potentially serious adverse side effects, this treatment is only indicated for patients with severe, widespread, atopic dermatitis that hasn't responded to other aggressive therapy.

>> **Hospitalization:** If your case of atopic dermatitis is extremely severe, your physician may need to remove you from environmental allergens, irritants, and emotional stress to effectively treat your unrelenting symptoms.

>> **Phosphodiesterase (PDE) inhibitors:** Crisaborole (Eucrisa) has broad spectrum anti-inflammatory activity by targeting the phosphodiesterase 4 (PDE4) enzyme that is a key regulator of inflammatory cytokine production. Blocking the overactive PDE4 enzymes within the skin cells helps to reduce the inflammation associated with eczema. Eucrisa is a prescription steroid-free ointment used on the skin and is approved in adults and children 3 months of age and older.

>> **Calcineurin inhibitors, tacrolimus (Protopic) and pimecrolimus (Elidel):** Researchers have developed ointments (Protopic) and creams (Elidel) that have been found to be effective in reducing or eliminating skin rashes in the majority of patients with atopic dermatitis who were tested. In contrast to topical corticosteroid preparations, tacrolimus and pimecrolimus have no potential to cause skin atrophy (thinning) and are highly effective therapies for atopic dermatitis. These topical medications, approved for treatment of atopic dermatitis, may potentially be of particular benefit in children, among whom an alternative to the chronic use of topical or oral corticosteroids would be extremely preferable. Elidel was recently approved for infants as young as three months of age, whereas Protopic is available in two strengths: 0.03% for ages two years and older and 0.1% for patients 16 years and older.

>> **Biologics:** Dupilumab (Dupixent), 6 months and older, and tralokinumab (Adbry, Adtralza), 12 years and older. These injectable treatments are targeted toward patients with moderate to severe atopic dermatitis whose disease isn't adequately controlled with topical prescription therapies. Dupilumab is a monoclonal antibody that inhibits interleukin-4 and interleukin-13, while tralokinumab, also a monoclonal antibody, selectively inhibits interleukin-13 only and is available in two dosages for aged 12–17 years and patients 18 years and older.

>> **Humanized monoclonal antibody:** Lebrikizumab (Ebglyss), a humanized monoclonal antibody also used for the treatment of atopic dermatitis was approved in 2023 only in the European Union in patients weighing

40kgs/88lbs. Lebrikizumab blocks IL-13, a cytokine involved in the inflammatory reaction associated with atopic dermatitis.

» **JAK inhibitors:** Upadacitinib (Rinvoq) and abrocitinib (Cibinqo) 12 years and older in the form of a once-a-day pill works by blocking certain signals inside the body that contribute to excess inflammation. It can lower the ability to fight infections and cause other side effects due to a suppressed immune system. Always check with your physician before starting a course of this medication.

Chapter **12**

Evaluating Contact Dermatitis

I f you just realized that the lush riverbank where you caught some rays yesterday was full of poison ivy, poison oak, or poison sumac, then this chapter is for you. Here, we include important information and tips on diag-nosing, treating, and avoiding the many manifestations of contact dermatitis that can occur in everyday life.

Contact dermatitis is a condition that occurs when the skin physically contacts an irritant or allergen that triggers a reaction, usually at the site of exposure. The reaction often produces inflammation, resulting in symptoms such as a skin rash, blistering, itching and burning sensations, and cracked or crusting areas of the skin. According to recent studies, contact dermatitis — in various forms — affects more than 10 percent of the U.S. population; and in the workplace, contact derma-titis accounts for almost one quarter of occupational disease cases, representing a significant cause of workplace disability.

Classifying Contact Dermatitis

Because allergens and irritants both cause contact dermatitis, the diseases are classified either as *allergic contact dermatitis* or *irritant contact dermatitis*. Each name refers to the types of triggers that cause your reactions, as we explain in this section. Based on historical, clinical, and patch-test findings (see the section "Diagnosing Contact Dermatitis" later in this chapter), approximately 80 percent of all contact dermatitis cases are due to irritants, while only 20 percent are directly triggered by allergens.

REMEMBER

The key to managing any form of contact dermatitis is identifying the irritants or allergens that affect you and avoiding or limiting contact with those substances, if possible.

Treatment for most cases of contact dermatitis involves using cold compresses and topical corticosteroid preparations for symptomatic relief. We provide more details on contact dermatitis relief in the section "Treating Contact Dermatitis" later in this chapter.

Irritant contact dermatitis

This condition, the result of direct physical injury to the skin, represents the vast majority of cases of contact dermatitis. Irritating or toxic man-made substances such as solvents, acids, or harsh soaps usually cause irritant contact dermatitis. In addition, direct skin contact with plants that possess chemically irritating sap, thorns, spines, nettles, and sharp-edged leaves — such as creeping spurge, poinsettias, cast bean, buttercup, and certain cacti — can also evoke symptoms of irritant contact dermatitis.

Unlike allergic contact dermatitis, the skin reaction that results from irritant contact dermatitis is nonallergic (*non-immunologic*) and usually begins shortly after (often within minutes) of your initial contact with the offending substance.

In some instances, symptoms occur because of repeated contact and long exposure to an irritating substance, such as detergent (in the case of *dishpan hands*). In fact, irritants are capable of causing contact dermatitis in anyone (whether you're allergic or nonallergic) if the irritants are applied against the skin in sufficient concentration for a long enough period of time.

Allergic contact dermatitis

In contrast with irritant contact dermatitis, allergic contact dermatitis only occurs in that smaller percentage of susceptible individuals who are sensitized to particular contact allergens and who in many cases have experienced prior sensitization.

While irritant reactions tend to occur within a few minutes of exposure to an offending substance, frequently case burning and pain, and are directly dependent on the dose of irritant to which a person is exposed, allergic contact dermatitis — which is due to a type 4 immunologic reaction (see Chapter 2) — typically appears 36 to 48 hours following exposure to the allergen, causes itching more often as a primary symptom, and can occur following exposure to much lower amounts of allergen compared with irritant dermatitis. That means that if you're highly allergic to a contact allergen, you can have a significant reaction even with exposure to only a small dose of the specific contact allergen. Many substances, such as the resin of *Toxicodendron* plants (poison ivy, poison oak, and poison sumac) as well as latex, formaldehyde, and nickel in the items that you use, wear, or come into contact with on a frequent basis, can trigger allergic reactions in sensitized individuals.

Often the terms allergic contact dermatitis and eczema are used interchangeably. Unlike atopic dermatitis and other atopic conditions — such as allergic rhinitis (hay fever), food allergies, and asthma, which can appear in various organs — symptoms of allergic contact dermatitis are local or *topical*, which means that these symptoms occur only where the allergen touches your skin. Indirect reactions can also occur if your hand or finger initially contacts an allergen and then spreads it to other parts of your body (see the "Identifying signs and symptoms" section later).

Understanding Allergic Contact Dermatitis Triggers

In contrast with atopic dermatitis, a family history of allergies doesn't play a role in determining whether you have a predisposition to developing allergic contact dermatitis. In fact, nonallergic people are just as likely to develop allergic contact dermatitis as those people who have other allergies. That's because the human immune system has two general ways of responding when it detects the presence of foreign organism or substances, including allergens:

>> **Humoral immunity:** Also known as *antibody response*, this process, which involves the production of IgE antibodies (which we explain in Chapter 2), is associated with allergic diseases such as atopic dermatitis, allergic rhinitis, food allergies, and certain drug allergies. The allergic reaction usually begins immediately or very soon after allergen exposure, may target different organs

of your body, and can range — depending on the type of exposure and your sensitivity level — from barely bothersome to life-threatening.

>> **Cell-mediated immunity (CMI):** This is the way the immune system responds in allergic contact dermatitis. Doctors also use the term *delayed hypersensitivity* (see Chapter 2) to describe this process, in which allergen contact results in an allergic reactions hours or even days after initial contact. (For example, you may not realize you've contacted poison ivy until your drive home from the weekend camping trip.) Although a delayed reaction is rarely life-threatening, it may take longer to subside or disappear than atopic-condition reactions in some cases. Because CMI allergic reactions don't involve the production of specific antibodies by the immune system, prick-puncture skin tests and allergy shots aren't effective diagnostic or treatment procedures when dealing with allergic contact dermatitis. (See Chapter 2 for more information regarding the different types of immunological reactions.)

A rash of allergens

Allergic contact dermatitis triggers abound throughout the modern world. At least 3,000 chemicals in use today can potentially trigger allergic contact dermatitis symptoms. For this reason, manufacturers are constantly testing new products prior to marketing — especially cosmetics, fragrances, and hair dyes — in an attempt to avoid introducing new items that may cause adverse allergic reactions.

Many of the organic and artificial substances and materials that people use in a wide variety of products and industries (agriculture, healthcare, manufacturing, and so on) can act as allergens if people become sensitized to them. For example, bank tellers and cashiers who constantly handle large amounts of cash can develop contact allergies to some of the chemicals and ink in bank notes and nickel in the coins that they handle. (Keep in mind, however, that bank tellers handle very large numbers of bills and coins all day long. The possibility that your teenagers may suddenly develop and allergy to the cash that you give them is less likely.)

If we listed all the substances, compounds, and products that potentially cause allergic contact dermatitis, we'd have to call this book *Heavy Book Lifting For Dummies*; that's how extensive the list would be. In the following sections, we provide you with a more concise and practical list of the most common chemicals and substances that can affect you.

Toxicodendron

The *Toxicodendron* family of plants, which includes poison ivy, poison oak, and poison sumac, is perhaps the most infamous source of allergic contact dermatitis cases and frequently causes streaky *lesions* (irritated reddening) developing on skin areas brushed by the plant. (Some physicians refer to this type of allergic contact dermatitis as *Rhus dermatitis*.) In fact, almost 85 percent of the U.S. population reacts to the resin from these plants. In the section "Poison Pointers: Making It Better" later in this chapter we give you more specific information on dealing with these plants.

Latex and other rubber compounds

Although poison ivy may make the headlines, you can find many more allergic contact dermatitis triggers without leaving your home, office, or school. For example, look around you; many items in your environment probably contain latex, which is the sap of the Brazilian rubber tree. Both the proteins in the natural tree sap and the chemicals that are added in the manufacturing process to the tree sap can trigger allergic contact dermatitis. Many synthetic rubber compounds can also act as allergic contact dermatitis triggers.

Current estimates are that between 1 to 6 percent of the general population in the United States experience sensitivity to latex and other rubber compounds. In fact, the percentages among healthcare workers are even higher in the range of 8 to 12 percent, which translates into about 1 to 2 million individuals working in the healthcare Industry.

Other common latex and synthetic rubber-containing items include

>> Office and school products, such as rubber bands and erasers

>> Athletic shoes and other sports equipment items (rubber handgrips on bicycles and tennis racquets, for example)

>> Baby and children's items, such as rubber toys, balloons, pacifiers, infant bottle nipples, and disposable diaper fasteners

>> Household items, including carpet backing, pillows, and cushions

>> Clothes — especially waterproof apparel, such as raincoats, galoshes and boots, rubber gloves, and the elastic in many types of underwear

>> Medical products (such as surgical gloves, face masks, adhesive bandages, hot water bottles, intravenous tubing, catheters, and syringes)

>> Contraceptives, such as condoms and diaphragms

TIP

For most of the products in the previous list, you can find nonlatex alternatives. For example, you can use gloves made of vinyl or Tactylon (a form of plastic) as a common substitute for latex gloves. However, if finding rubber-free products is expensive, impractical, or inconvenient, you may want to consider *patch testing* (see the "Patch testing" section later in this chapter) to confirm that natural rubber is actually triggering your dermatitis. Likewise, you may also want to check whether other rubber chemicals such as those in the thiuram group (commonly used in adhesives and disinfectants) or those in the thiourea group (used in detergents and photocopy paper) may also trigger your skin reaction due to allergic contact dermatitis.

Many fungicides, wood preservatives, anticorrosion agents, surgical dressings, plastics, and adhesives contain nonlatex rubber compounds that can also trigger allergic contact dermatitis. These substances often affect workers in health, plastics, chemical, and agriculture industries.

WARNING

In addition to triggering symptoms of allergic contact dermatitis, *natural rubber latex* (NRL) proteins can attach to the corn starch powder that is used in some latex gloves and can subsequently trigger immediate and serious systemic allergic reactions in susceptible individuals. Physicians refer to this reaction as *Type 1 IgE-mediated immediate hypersensitivity* (see Chapter 2). This type of systemic reaction occurs from inhaling latex allergen particles in the air, affecting organs other than the skin. Symptoms can include runny nose, sneezing, itchy eyes, scratchy throat, coughing, and in severe cases, wheezing and difficulty breathing, similar to an asthma attack. Widespread hives an angioedema (deep swellings) can also result, possibly progressing to *anaphylaxis* (a potentially life-threatening reaction that affects many organs simultaneously) in some individuals.

SEE YOUR DOCTOR

If you notice these sorts of nasal or respiratory symptoms when you're exposed to latex, have your physician check it out. You may be suffering from a more serious type of allergic condition. A history of hand dermatitis from wearing rubber gloves may also be a warning sign of latex sensitivity.

TIP

If you've experienced a previous systemic reaction to latex, you should take active measures to avoid future exposure to the substance. Make sure that you notify (in writing) all your healthcare providers — including your dentist and pharmacist — of your immediate hypersensitivity to latex. We also advise you to remind these professionals of your allergy every time you visit their offices.

If your occupation (in the United States) exposes you to latex — for example, by using latex gloves (as a healthcare worker) or by breathing latex dust as a result of being directly involved in the manufacturing process — you should read recent advisories from the U.S. Occupational Safety and Health Administration (OSHA), which provide you and your employer with guidelines on how to reduce unnecessary exposure to NRL proteins on the job. OSHA bulletins are usually posted in workplaces and can be requested from your local state OSHA office or from the U.S. Department of Labor, Occupational Safety & Health Administration, Office of Public Affairs Room N3647, 200 Constitution Avenue, Washington, D.C., 20210; (202) 693-1999; www.osha.gov/.

Nickel

Remember what we told you about cashiers who develop allergen sensitivities because of the number of coins that they handle? (See the introductory text in this chapter.) The source of the bank tellers' allergic reaction is nickel, a metallic element that you can find in many of the objects that you touch in your daily life. Allergic reactions to nickel can include an eczema-type rash, itching, and hive-like skin eruptions. The following is more than five cents' worth of important information about nickel:

» At least 10 percent of the U.S. population suffers from a sensitivity to nickel. This sensitivity is ten times more common in women than in men, because women usually wear more costume jewelry than men and generally start wearing it at an earlier age. However, men are more likely to suffer from occupational *contact* dermatitis involving nickel because they're more likely than women to work in fields such as mining, engineering, construction, and as jewelers.

» Ear piercing plays a significant role in the development of an allergic condition from nickel exposure. In many cases, people who suffer from a nickel allergy display scars or eczema around their ear lobes, because many earrings and earring posts contain nickel.

» Other forms of jewelry that contain nickel can also produce allergic skin reactions, such as clasps, fasteners, belt buckles, buttons and rivets on jeans, snaps, and eyeglass frames. Your perspiration leaches nickel out of these objects, allowing the skin to absorb the element and trigger a rash. A common nickel reaction often occurs on the wrist, under your watch.

» Coins, pocketknives, keys, and cigarette lighters and cases that you carry in your pants pockets can produce skin eruptions on your thighs.

» Mascara, eyeshadow, and eye pencils often contain nickel and can therefore cause facial dermatitis in sensitized individuals.

» Other typical sources of nickel contact include door handles, doorknobs, drawer handles, bicycle handlebars, show buckles, kitchen utensils and cookware, scissors, knitting needles, umbrellas, and many stationery items such as pens, pencils, and paper clips.

TIP

If you're sensitive to nickel, one solution may be to wear only jewelry and accessories with higher gold content. (You can tell people that you're allergic to cheap jewelry!) We also suggest wearing a protective layer between your skin and any items that contain nickel. For example, try carrying items such as coins, keys, pocketknives, and so on in a pouch or other enclosure that prevents nickel from leaching onto your skin.

Paraphenylenediamine (PPD)

Paraphenylenediamine (PPD) is a chemical that manufacturers use in dyes, particularly for darker shades of hair color, fur, and clothing. If you suffer from a sensitivity to this chemical, you many also suffer cross-reactivity (see Chapter 2) to related chemicals, such as those in stamp-pad ink, sulfa drugs, color film developer, and epoxy resin. Here are some key points to keep in mind about PPD and allergic contact dermatitis:

>> Hairdressers can easily develop allergies to PPD. In fact, most hair dye labels advise hairdressers to perform patch tests before using their products.

>> If you're allergic to PPD, make sure that you inform your health providers — especially your pharmacist — because some people with this allergy may also react to sulfa drugs, such as sulfisoxazole (Gantrisin) and trimethoprim-sulfamethoxazole (Bactrim, Septra).

>> Because of cross-reactivity, topical and injected anesthetics such as Benzocaine and some other so-called -caines (Novocain, Nesacaine, Pontocaine, Butyn, Butesin) can also trigger allergic contact dermatitis symptoms if you possess PPD sensitivities. Other common -caines, such as Xylocaine, Marcaine, Sensorcaine, Carbocaine, and Nupercaine aren't as likely to cross-react with PPD.

>> Sunscreens that contain para-aminobenzoic acid (PABA) can cause allergic contact dermatitis because of a cross-reactivity with PPD or can trigger photoallergic contact dermatitis, a related condition that we explain in "Photoallergic contact dermatitis (PACD)" later in this chapter. In both cases, we advise using sunscreens labeled "PF," which stands for PABA-free (How's that for technical terminology?)

Ethylenediamine (EDA)

Ethylenediamine (EDA) has been used as a stabilizer in prescription topical anti-infective medications such as Mycolog Cream (often used for treating diaper rash) and similar generic products. EDA is also an ingredient in asthma medications such as aminophylline and in antihistamines such as hydroxyzine (Atarax), antazoline (Vasocon A), and mepyramine (Pyrilamine). Also keep the following facts in mind about EDA:

>> Many people use Mycolog II Cream and similar generics to treat fungal skin infections. However, the EDA in these types of preparations can act as a sensitizer. Asthma patients who are subsequently given intravenous forms of aminophylline (theophylline EDA), which doctors occasionally use for treatment of respiratory symptoms, can experience systemic reactions,

including systemic contact dermatitis (widespread rashes over the entire body) and even life-threatening systemic allergic reactions. (See Chapter 16 for more information on adverse drug reactions.)

>> Pharmacists who frequently handle antibiotic compounds can develop sensitivities to EDA that can lead to systemic reactions if they take the antibiotics internally.

Formalin

As the liquid form of the gas formaldehyde, formalin can cause allergic contact dermatitis on the hands. A wide variety of products, such as the following, commonly use formalin:

>> Drip-dry, permanent press, and water-repellent garments, tanned leather and furs, as well as dry cleaning and potting fluids, include formalin.

>> Shampoos, soaps, underarm deodorants, bath preparations, mascara, and so on.

>> Antifreeze and anticorrosive agents.

>> Paints, paint removers, varnishes, and polishes.

>> Disinfectants, detergents, and household and industrial cleaners.

>> Paper, ink, and photographic developers.

>> Insecticides, fumigants, and agricultural chemicals.

Potassium dichromate

Chromates can cause allergic contact dermatitis on the hands and fingers of construction workers, who expose themselves to this metal in cement, mortar, plaster, rust removers, boiler cleaner and even in the leather gloves they might be wearing. In some cases, systemic reactions can also occur if workers inhale dust from work materials. Some sensitized individuals experience rashes on the tops of their feet because of contact with the potassium dichromate that manufacturers use to tan shoes.

Other allergic contact dermatitis conditions

In certain circumstances, the allergic contact dermatitis triggers that we discuss in the section "A rash of allergens" in this chapter (yes, that was the short list) can also cause related types of allergic skin conditions in sensitized individuals. In some cases, allergic contact dermatitis results from additional factors such as interaction with sunlight, overuse of topical medications, or even contact with your partner. In addition, urticaria (hives) can result from a contact reaction.

Photoallergic contact dermatitis (PACD)

No, photoallergic contact dermatitis (PACD) isn't the result of looking at a photograph of yourself taken on a bad hair day that makes your skin crawl. PACD is a rash or eczema condition that occurs from an interaction (known as *persistent light reaction*) between ultraviolet (UV) light (sunlight) and topical products that contain substances to which you're sensitized. These products can include

>> **PABA:** You can frequently find this substance in sunscreens. However, using sunscreens with PABA can lead to a rash on the face or other skin areas. Because doctors advise using sunscreens to protect your skin from overexposure to UV rays, we recommend always using PABA-free (PF) sunscreens such as PreSun, Ti-Screen, Shade Sunblock, and many others. Check the labels on sunscreens that you want to use or ask your pharmacist for advice on these products.

>> **Musk ambrette:** This synthetic chemical, used mostly in men's aftershave and cologne, can cause an eczema-type rash in reaction with sunlight. If you're sensitive to this substance, we advise using only fragrance-free products.

>> *Topical antibacterials: Sulfa drugs and topical antihistamines such as diphenhydramine cream (Benadryl) can also trigger PACD.* If you treat a skin condition with these products and you experience eczema reactions when you're in the sun, ask your physician to recommend alternative medications. If they give you a prescription for topical or oral antibiotics, they should warn you against sun exposure while taking the medication. (See Chapter 16 for more information on drug interactions.)

Connubial contact dermatitis

Connubial contact dermatitis, also sometimes called *consort contact dermatitis*, applies mostly to couples, as the name suggests. While we're certainly in favor of sharing as a basis for a healthy relationship, sharing everything isn't wise. Although allergies aren't contagious, sharing personal hygiene products and medications can expose you and your significant other to allergy triggers that many not affect the other person.

Connubial contact dermatitis often results from sharing deodorant, hair products, contact lens solutions, skin products, intimate devices, and other items that come into contact with porous parts of the body (including genital areas). Outbreaks of this type of contact dermatitis usually results in eczema (and sometimes hives) on the face, neck, hands, or genitals.

Contact urticaria

Urticaria is the medical term for hives. Hives can erupt as a result of allergic and nonallergic reactions to a variety of irritants and allergens. In Chapter 13, we cover hives that erupt because of systemic reactions to foods, insect bites and stings, and drugs, as well as light, water, temperature extremes, and stress and exercise. That chapter also gives you helpful tips on diagnosing and treating hives and angioedema (a related form of skin swelling).

Physicians classify contact forms of hives as *nonallergic* and *allergic*. The following list focuses on the two most common forms of contact hives:

>> **Nonallergic contact urticaria:** This form of hives can affect people who aren't sensitized to an allergy trigger or irritant. With this disease, hives can erupt soon after your skin contacts substances such as insect and spider hairs, alcohol, sodium benzoate, acetic acid, sorbic acid, balsam of Peru, cobalt chloride, and even an over-the-counter topical antibiotic such as bacitracin (Betadine).

>> **Allergic contact urticaria:** With this form of hives, the hives may erupt as a result of skin contact with triggering substances in raw potatoes, fish, and liver (yet another reason not to like liver!) as well as substances in antibiotics, natural rubber, epoxy, and treated wood.

Systemic contact dermatitis

If you overuse topical medications (antibacterial creams, ointments, or topical antihistamines), your skin may absorb some of the allergens that these products can contain. Your immune system may then produce antibodies against those allergens. If you subsequently receive an oral or injected form of the medication to which your body became sensitized as a result of previous allergic dermatitis, severe systemic reactions can potentially occur (as we explain in the "Ethylenediamine (EDA)" section earlier in this chapter).

TIP

Because your body can become sensitized to allergens in skin care products, we advise against applying creams, lotions, and ointments for every minor skin irritation, rash, or itch that occurs. In many cases, minor skin problems may respond well to simple remedies such as cold compresses and commonsense avoidance practices.

For example, if you develop a rash during hot weather and you've been wearing tight-fitting clothes, slip into something looser and more comfortable. You'll probably perspire less, which means that fewer of the irritants and allergens that may be present in your garments will leach out into your skin. Looser clothing probably also means less direct rubbing or pressure on the area where the rash has developed, which should help the inflammation to subside if it's not the result of a more serious condition.

SEE YOUR DOCTOR

Apply cold compresses before resorting to topical medications, unless your condition lingers, rapidly worsens, or spreads; or if you're experiencing symptoms of a systemic reaction. In those cases, we strongly advise seeing a physician. Depending on the nature, extent, and severity of your condition, you may be referred also to a dermatologist or allergist for further evaluation and treatment.

Diagnosing Contact Dermatitis

Often, the cause of your condition is obvious. However, because most people constantly come into contact with so many potential irritants and allergens — as ingredients or compounds in a multitude of products at home, work, or school — identifying the true cause of your dermatitis may challenge your physician at times. In fact, you and your physician may need to thoroughly examine and investigate many aspects of your life to determine what causes your skin condition.

Diagnosing your skin condition may also require a special form of skin testing known as a *patch test.* Patch testing can help your physician determine whether your dermatitis is due to allergy and which specific allergens trigger this type of allergic reaction. (We discuss patch testing in the section "Patch testing" later in this chapter.)

Identifying symptoms and signs

Characteristic signs of allergic contact dermatitis include a red rash, swollen pimples, blisters, and itchy skin. These symptoms may appear hours to days after your skin contacts an allergen, and they usually develop where the allergen touches your skin. As you may expect, the part of your skin that touches the allergen usually shows the most severe inflammation. Very often, the outline of your rash and the location on your body where it appears can provide your doctor with important clues in diagnosing the specific cause of your allergic contact dermatitis (see Figure 12-1).

REMEMBER

Your hands can also transmit allergens to other parts of your body, where the rash and other symptoms develop most noticeably. For example, although allergens or irritants in mascara, eye shadow, eyeliner, and other cosmetics can often cause eyelid eczema, an allergen in fingernail polish may cause the problem in some cases. If you're sensitized to an allergen in fingernail polish and you rub your eyes, the rash may appear on both your upper and lower eyelids.

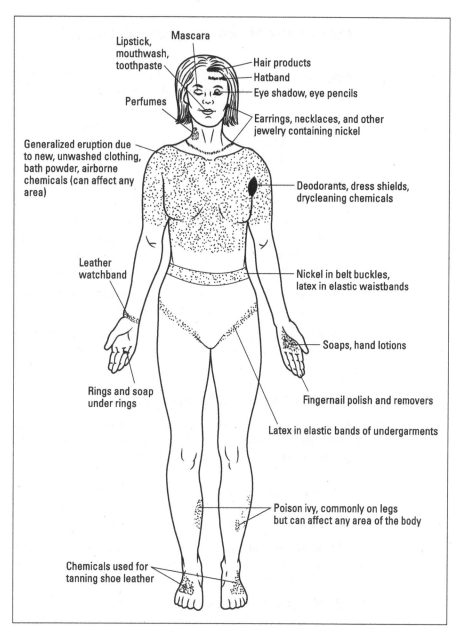

Lipstick, mouthwash, toothpaste

Mascara

Hair products

Hatband

Eye shadow, eye pencils

Perfumes

Earrings, necklaces, and other jewelry containing nickel

Generalized eruption due to new, unwashed clothing, bath powder, airborne chemicals (can affect any area)

Deodorants, dress shields, drycleaning chemicals

Leather watchband

Nickel in belt buckles, latex in elastic waistbands

Soaps, hand lotions

Rings and soap under rings

Fingernail polish and removers

Latex in elastic bands of undergarments

Poison ivy, commonly on legs but can affect any area of the body

Chemicals used for tanning shoe leather

FIGURE 12-1: Common areas and causes of contact dermatitis.

© John Wiley & Sons, Inc.

More ways of skinning your dermatitis

The extent and severity of your allergic contact dermatitis reaction can also depend on other factors that you and your doctor need to consider in the diagnostic process, as we explain in the following points:

>> Skin conditions can coexist. In some cases, allergens in topical products that you use to treat eczema caused by atopic dermatitis can trigger allergic contact dermatitis.

>> If your skin is already inflamed or irritated, it may be more susceptible to contact dermatitis.

>> The sensitivity levels of your skin's different areas can vary greatly. The thinner the skin, the greater the absorption of contact allergens. For this reason, in general, your eyelids, neck, and genital areas are the most sensitive, while palms, soles of feet, and your scalp are more resistant to outbreaks.

>> More than half of all cases of contact dermatitis (whether allergic or nonallergic) affect the hands, due to increased exposure.

>> If enough allergens remain on your skin following an initial reaction, flare-ups can sometimes occur weeks to years after exposure.

Variations on a skin disease

Because eczema is a common symptom of many dermatitis diseases, your physician also needs to consider other possible causes of your symptoms. Other potential causes of eczema could include the following medical conditions:

>> **Seborrheic dermatitis:** This condition usually involves eczema around the scalp and nose. With infants, if the top of the head, armpit, and diaper area show signs of eczema, seborrheic dermatitis is the likely cause.

>> **Atopic dermatitis:** As we explain in Chapter 11, this condition often involves a systemic reaction to allergens that can also trigger other allergies such as allergic rhinitis. Physicians also often link atopic dermatitis to food allergies.

>> **Phototoxic dermatitis (PICD):** This nonallergic condition, sometimes called exaggerated sunburn, often results from an interaction between intense sunlight and topical exposure to chemicals in coal tar products, sulfa drugs, and certain dyes. Substances in citrus fruits and celery can also act as precipitants of this condition. Bartenders and other beverage servers who work outside and squeeze limes and lemons into drinks while exposed to intense sunlight can experience forms of PICD (sometimes called *phytodermatitis*), often two to three days after exposure. Symptoms usually include rash, skin swelling, pimples, and blisters.

>> **Irritant contact dermatitis:** As we mention at the beginning of this chapter, this form of contact dermatitis is nonallergic, but symptoms can appear virtually identical to those of allergic contact dermatitis. Irritant contact dermatitis occurs frequently because of the wide variety of substances in our modern world — especially in the workplace — that can irritate the skin.

The skinny on your skin condition

SEE YOUR DOCTOR

A careful, thorough medical history evaluation is vital to diagnosing the correct cause of your dermatitis condition. Therefore, your physician may inquire in great detail about many aspects of your life. They need this level of information to narrow the range of potential contact allergens and irritants, from the thousands that you're exposed to every day to the most likely suspects. Try to answer your physician as thoroughly as possible about subjects such as

>> Your symptoms, your general health, other conditions, and illnesses you may have suffered, and your family medical history

>> Your home, work, or school environments

>> Your important clues to the nature of your condition in descriptions of your hobbies, recreational activities, and the types of clothing that you wear

>> The time and place when your symptoms appear can also help your doctor with your diagnosis

TIP

In some cases, your symptoms may subside before you get to see your physician. In such instances, you may want to take a photo on your smartphone of your skin condition (if practical) to show the extent and severity of your dermatitis.

Patch testing

The most important medical procedure that physicians use in confirming the diagnosis of allergic contact dermatitis is patch testing. This test can also be used to establish the diagnosis of irritant contact dermatitis.

The patch test involves applying patches that contain small, diluted amounts of suspected allergens directly to the skin. Your physician uses the results of this test to see whether the applied allergens have caused a small area of allergic contact dermatitis. Think of the patch test process as a miniature reproduction of your skin condition. In most cases, common contact allergens are placed on small aluminum discs and then taped onto the surface of your skin so that several patches with different allergens can all be applied in rows at the same time.

REMEMBER

Your physician should only perform patch testing after they take a thorough medical examination of your condition and perform a complete physical examination. These procedures enable your physician to focus on testing the most likely suspects from a list of more than 3,000 substances that trigger allergic contact dermatitis.

WARNING

Never agree to a patch test if your dermatitis is severe or widespread. Likewise, your physician should instruct you to immediately remove any patch that causes severe itching or discomfort.

SEE YOUR DOCTOR

In some cases, they may ask you to bring materials from your home, work, or school that may contain suspected contact allergy triggers to use in your patch test.

Patch testing is generally done on your upper back in rows, directly onto skin that is free of any signs of dermatitis. In some cases, doctors may alternatively apply patch tests to the upper, outer arm. Each patch contains one suspected allergen, with a corresponding number or letter on the patch that identifies the test substance. The number and types of substances that may be administered in a patch test depend on what your physician thinks might be causing your skin problem.

Your physician will instruct you to keep the patches in place for at least 48 hours and to avoid wetting them (for example, by taking a shower) during this time period. In addition, while the patches are in place, your physician will most likely ask you to refrain from strenuous sports or any other types of heavy work or recreational activity that could result in significant perspiration (yes, you can be a couch potato, but only for two days!). Your physician will also usually ask you to return to the office 48 hours after the patch tests have been applied and will remove the patches and interpret the results of the test at that time.

A positive reaction to the suspected allergen produces small-scale symptoms that mimic your dermatitis condition. Because positive tests can continue producing reactions, these patch test sites are frequently reexamined after 72 hours. Some positive reactions may not occur for 96 hours (four days, in case you're counting) or even one week, as is often the case when testing for neomycin (Neosporin ointment), a common topical antibiotic.

However, because positive reactions can also indicate the presence of other allergic sensitivities — unrelated to your current dermatitis — the patch test results should also correlate with your physical examination and medical history to identify the suspected allergen more conclusively. Experienced physicians know you don't treat the lab results, you treat the patient. Incidental findings that don't correlate with the patient's medical history require further evaluation by a specialist.

Treating Contact Dermatitis

The most effective way of dealing with contact dermatitis in any form — and preventing future episodes — is avoiding whatever causes the problem.

TIP

If avoiding the trigger isn't possible or practical, treating the rash and other types of dermatitis outbreaks with simple home remedies can provide effective relief from mild symptoms. The following sections identify ways you can treat contact dermatitis.

Doing it yourself

If you experience a limited episode of allergic contact dermatitis, try using cold water compresses. You can make these compresses from any clean, soft, smooth cotton material. Use cool (not hot) tap water or a solution that your physician recommends, such as Burow's solution, to dampen the compress, and then apply it to your inflamed area. Leave the compress in place for half an hour before removing it. Repeat this procedure two to six times a day, depending on your physician's specific advice.

SEE YOUR
DOCTOR

If your physician also prescribes a topical corticosteroid cream, such as hydrocortisone, your compresses facilitate absorption of the cream and can also enhance its anti-inflammatory effect.

In some cases, they may advise you to only use compresses until the skin condition begins to subside. They may then direct you to discontinue using the compresses and to start applying only the topical corticosteroid cream.

TIP

Be nice to your skin. You must keep your skin clean but avoid using harsh soaps because they damage your skin's natural protective layer. Likewise, don't overdo bathing (even with gentle soaps), because doing so can dry out your skin, increasing the chance of contacting irritants and allergens that cause inflammation. We recommend frequently (three to four times per day) lubricating your affected area with a lotion or ointment that your doctor recommends. As we explain in Chapter 11, you also need to apply moisturizers immediately after bathing and avoid drying off briskly. Gently using a soft towel to pat yourself dry retains vital moisture.

Turning to medication

The products that physicians usually prescribe to relieve allergic contact dermatitis symptoms include topical corticosteroids and oral antihistamines. In cases of severe symptoms, your physician may prescribe oral systemic corticosteroids. Likewise, if you suffer from infected skin lesions, they may also prescribe an appropriate course of oral antibiotics.

Topical corticosteroids

Topical corticosteroid products are available in various strengths. Your physician determines the most appropriate form and dosage for you, however, because different areas of your body may require different potencies, depending on the extent and severity of your dermatitis, physicians generally make low potency hydrocortisone creams their first choice for the treatment of mild allergic contact dermatitis symptoms. Low potency hydrocortisone creams are also the only products that we recommend using on your face or on the skin of infants and young children. Areas of thicker skin, such as the palms of your hands and the soles of your feet require stronger topical corticosteroid creams. Prolonged use of very high potency topical applications is associated with serious side effects such as systemic absorption and thinning of the affected skin. Therefore, you should use the least potent topical corticosteroid whenever possible. (See Chapter 11 for the potency ratings of common topical corticosteroids.)

WARNING

Usually, your physician will advise you to apply the product evenly over the affected area. In more severe cases, they may advise using an occlusive (barrier) dressing such as plastic wrap to prevent evaporation of the topical preparation and to enhance its penetration into the skin. Although this can be a valuable technique in the short term, using occlusive dressing for an extensive period can increase the risk of local or systemic side effects from the application of topical corticosteroids. Make sure that you follow the product instructions and your physician's recommendations, because topical corticosteroids can cause serious adverse side effects if you don't use them properly.

Oral antihistamines

Oral antihistamines can often relieve the itching symptoms that frequently aggravate dermatitis conditions. Depending on the severity of your symptoms, your physician may prescribe a less-sedating (Zyrtec) or a nonsedating second-generation antihistamine such as Allegra or Claritin. Or they may prescribe an over-the-counter (OTC) sedating antihistamine if you can't sleep at night because of the inflammation and intense itching. However, you should be aware that the sedative side effects of these products may persist during the day and if you suffer from restless leg syndrome, it can make symptoms worse.

Severe cases

If you suffer from a particularly acute and extensive allergic reaction, your physician may prescribe a short course of oral corticosteroids, such as prednisone.

In cases where bacterial infection occurs — usually from scratching itchy rashes and lesions — we recommend using only oral antibiotics to clear the infection. Don't apply topical antihistamine and antibiotic products because these drugs can actually aggravate the condition by provoking an allergic reaction if a patient is already sensitized to the substances in these products.

For the Love of Ivy — Dealing with These Poison Plants

Poison ivy, poison oak, and poison sumac are native to many parts of North America and are widespread throughout the continent. The leaves of these poison plants contain *urushiol*, an *oleoresin* (oily resin). Contacting the leaves of these plants, in most people who are sensitized to this oleoresin, can cause blisters and a characteristic, streaky red rash with linear lesions on skin areas of the skin brushed by the plant. (Because poison ivy is the most prevalent of these plants, we refer to it alone in the rest of this section.)

Noticing resin reactions

The first exposure to urushiol is what sensitizes most people, but that exposure usually isn't enough to trigger a reaction. It usually takes significant subsequent contact for the symptoms to appear. Most people break out after a second major exposure to poison ivy or after several minor contacts, with symptoms usually occurring within two days.

Toxic transfers

Skin eruptions from poison ivy contact commonly result from the direct exposure of your bare skin to the plants while camping or hiking in the woods. However, other sources of exposure can include

>> **Animals:** Pets or other animals (who usually don't break out) that roam outdoors and carry the resin in their fur.

>> **Clothing:** Resin can stick to clothes and then transfer to people who touch the garments.

>> **Firewood:** If poison ivy grows around your woodpile, or if you gather firewood in areas with poison ivy, the resin may stick on the logs and transfer onto your hands or clothes.

>> **Gardening:** Performing yard work in areas with prevalent poison ivy can cause major resin exposure. For example, cleaning out lawn mower clippings can involve contact with urushiol if poison ivy grows in the grass that you mow. Poison ivy resin can also stick to garden tools, such as clippers, hedge trimmers, and rakes.

>> **Smoke:** If you burn any of these poison plants, the smoke can trigger reactions if you're especially sensitive to the allergens. Tiny droplets of the oleoresin in the smoke can potentially come into contact with your body and trigger a reaction that may include symptoms affecting your eyes and skin.

Don't scratch that itch

REMEMBER

Poison ivy skin conditions themselves aren't really contagious. Frequently the condition appears to spread to new areas of your body for several days after the initial outbreak. Contrary to popular belief, the fluid in blisters, rashes, and lesions doesn't contain the triggering allergen. Instead, the reason you may continue to experience outbreaks of poison ivy dermatitis is due to the different rates of absorption on the oleoresin by different parts of your body and the degree to which those areas were initially exposed.

WARNING

However, in some cases, if you don't thoroughly clean and remove all the oleoresin from your hands — and especially from under your fingernails — then you may in fact spread the allergen with your fingers. This can occur by scratching unaffected areas around your existing blisters, thus triggering new eruptions. You could even potentially spread the oleoresin to other individuals (perhaps giving new meaning to the term "nailing them," don't you think?). In addition, scratching your own lesions, blisters, or rashes can also result in skin infections from any bacteria that may reside on your hands.

Steering clear of poison problems

Avoiding all contact with poison plant is the easiest way to prevent exposure to the allergens that they contain. If you know that poison ivy grows on your property, you may want to consider killing it, as long as you can avoid exposure to its resin while doing so. Consider hiring a person who isn't sensitive to poison ivy to clean out the plants or do your yardwork. In addition, although poison ivy may be dormant in the winter, the dried vines still contain active oleoresin that can potentially trigger allergic contact dermatitis.

Some people with sensitivity to urushiol may also experience *cross-reactivity* (see Chapter 14) to the peel of mango fruit and the oil from the shell of cashew nuts. The appearance of a topical reaction after peeling mangos is the most common reaction, but more serious systemic symptoms, including nausea, vomiting, and diarrhea, can result if peelings contaminate the meat of the mango. However, mango that has not been contaminated by the peelings can be eaten without difficulty. (Let someone else peel it!)

Leaves of three, let them be

One of the best ways of avoiding contact with poison ivy and other related plants is to recognize their appearance. The easiest way to identify these plants is to look for the characteristic three-leaf cluster, hence the old saying, "Leaves of three, let it be." However, in winter, poison ivy loses its leaves and is less recognizable, so making yourself aware of the plant's possible locations can also help you avoid their resin's wrath.

Protecting yourself

You can lessen your chances of poison ivy contact by making sure that you expose your skin as little as possible when you're outside in areas where poison plants may grow. You can minimize exposure by following these suggestions:

» Wear clothing that covers as much of your skin as possible. In warmer weather, wear looser-filling garments and fabrics that breathe. Following these guidelines can help you stay comfortable and avoid the temptation to take off your clothing articles to keep cool.

» Use barrier creams such as Stokogard, Ivy Block, and Ivy Shield that can provide some protection for exposed areas of your skin. However, check with your physician before relying on these products because they can lose their effectiveness from perspiration, scratching, and abrasion. These products may not work for you if you plan to play or work extensively in areas where poison ivy exposure is a possibility.

Poison Pointers: Making It Better

If you think you've come into contact with poison ivy or other related poison plants, use these tips to help stop the spread of infection:

» Wash off any part of your skin that you may have exposed. If you wash off your skin within 5 to 30 minutes after contact — depending on your exposure and sensitivity levels to the plant — you may avoid developing a reaction. Soap and water work best to wash off the allergens, but sometimes even water alone can remove much of the plant resin that triggers your allergic contact dermatitis reaction. If water isn't immediately available, wash as soon as you can to minimize the extent of your reaction.

» Carefully remove and wash (or dry clean as indicated) your clothes, including gloves and shoes, as soon as possible to minimize spreading the resin to other parts of your body or to other people around you.

» If you camp, wash any gear — blankets, towels, sleeping bags, tents — that may have contacted the poison plants.

» To relieve reaction symptoms, apply cold, wet compresses — using a clean, soft uncontaminated cloth — to the inflamed areas of your skin. Calamine lotion, Burow's solution, and cool showers can also help relieve itching.

» If your face or genital areas are affected, or if your rash is widespread, see a physician as soon as possible. In severe cases, usually when 20 percent or more of the body is affected, they may prescribe a short course of oral prednisone.

Chapter **13**

Evaluating Hives and Angioedema

H ere's the rub on hives and angioedema: All that itches and erupts isn't allergic. Allergists see many patients with hives and *angioedema* (deep swellings) because almost a third of the U.S. population suffers at some point from these skin conditions and because most people assume that these itchy eruptions result from allergies.

REMEMBER

For the most part, however, that assumption is a myth. Allergic reactions trigger only some cases of hives and angioedema, whereas a variety of other causes (which we describe in this chapter) trigger the majority of eruptions. Hives and angioedema are the subject of many myths and mistaken assumptions, as illustrated in the following list:

» **I'm breaking out because of my nerves.** If this myth were true, we'd all break out during rush hour, school exams, or when trying to figure out how to pay our children's college tuition. Anxiety and other psychological factors may aggravate hives, but many other illnesses can also worsen when you're under a lot of stress.

» **Hives are a minor problem, and they only bother me temporarily.** Hives may bother some people only temporarily, but hives can also develop into a chronic condition that lasts several months or years. A persistent hives outbreak can also signal a serious underlying medical disorder, such as an infectious or rheumatoid disease, which may worsen if you and your physician don't diagnose, treat, and manage it appropriately.

WARNING

» **Only prescription drugs like penicillin cause hives or angioedema.** This statement is simply untrue. In fact, plain old everyday nonprescription aspirin is one of the most common causes of hives. Contrary to what you may expect — because hives and angioedema are inflammatory conditions and aspirin is an anti-inflammatory drug — you shouldn't, under any circumstances, take aspirin or related anti-inflammatory medications to relieve hives and angioedema. This rule also applies to nonsteroidal anti-inflammatory drugs (NSAIDs), most of which contain ibuprofen (Advil, Motrin), ketoprofen (Actron, Orudis), or naproxen (Aleve) as active ingredients. Also, avoid combination pain relievers that include any of these active ingredients.

» **My hives and angioedema are isolated disorders.** Physicians increasingly consider these conditions as possible symptoms of larger and potentially more serious underlying problems. As a result, more physicians are taking a global approach to the diagnosis and treatment of hives and angioedema. If your physician can't precisely determine the cause of your eruptions, you should seek appropriate consultation with a specialist (an allergist or a dermatologist) to help diagnose and manage your condition more effectively, as well as to make sure that you're not at risk for a more serious disorder.

REMEMBER

Although allergic triggers play important roles in some *acute* (rapid onset) forms of hives and angioedema, in many instances — particularly with chronic (long-term) hives — the causes of outbreaks aren't clear and appear to be unrelated to allergies. Most chronic hives and angioedema cases go undiagnosed. Your physician may refer to undiagnosed types of disorders as *idiopathic*, which means "of unknown cause." (It doesn't mean that they feel like an idiot for not identifying the source of your ailment.) Therefore, since the vast majority of the cause remains undiscovered, we use the term chronic idiopathic angioedema and urticaria which is an officially recognized diagnosis by both government and insurance companies. Fortunately, almost all cases can be well treated and the symptoms safely controlled.

Understanding Hives: Nettlesome Conditions

The medical term for hives is *urticaria*, from the Latin word *Urtica*, which means *nettles*. Indeed, the hallmark of hives is an outbreak of stinging, itchy welts, often resembling inflamed mosquito bites or the result of a close encounter between a thorny bush and your skin. These welts can worsen if you scratch them, and they may develop into *lesions* (a localized area of affected skin). The lesions can grow and run together into large areas, especially if you keep scratching them. Here we delve deeper into hives.

Classifying hives

Physicians classify most cases of hives either as acute urticaria or chronic urticaria. In case of *acute urticaria*, hives erupt quickly after exposure to trigger allergens or irritants or even without a known trigger. The outbreaks often subside within two hours and rarely last longer than 24 hours in one area. The disorder usually disappears within six to ten weeks.

Chronic spontaneous urticaria (CSU) involves persistently recurring eruptions of hives that last longer than 6 weeks. Allergens rarely seem to trigger chronic urticaria, and in most cases, the causes are difficult, if not impossible, to determine.

Focusing on other aspects

Consider the following about acute and chronic forms of hives:

>> Children and young adults generally experience most of the acute urticaria cases.

>> Upper respiratory viral infections, such as the common cold, are the most common infectious trigger of acute urticaria in children.

>> Food allergies cause a larger number of acute urticaria cases in children than in adults.

>> CSU is more frequent among the middle-aged, especially women.

>> More than one-third of patients who experience CSU for more than six months suffer recurring outbreaks of hives for at least ten years.

WARNING

>> Hive eruptions that persist in the same place on your skin for more than 24 hours may suggest symptoms of a more serious underlying condition, *urticarial vasculitis*. (See the section "Urticarial vasculitis and other systemic conditions" later in this chapter.)

Getting under Your Skin: Angioedema

In the previous section, we explain some Latin to help explain urticaria. At the risk of turning this book into *Ancient Languages For Dummies*, here's some Greek for you: *angeion* means "vessel" and *edema* translates to "swelling." Hence *angioedema*, the medical term that refers to a skin condition similar to hives. The main difference between hives and angioedema is that the inflammation from angioedema extends into deeper tissues, resulting in a characteristic swelling of the skin.

REMEMBER

Here are more key points that you need to keep in mind about angioedema:

>> Angioedema occurs in deeper skin layers, where fewer mast cells and sensory nerve endings reside. Therefore, the lesions cause little or no itching, and the swelling more often produces painful or burning sensations.

>> Angioedema may involve any part of the body. However, it affects the lips, eyelids, tongue, and genitalia more frequently. (These parts of your body have thinner skin and more blood circulation closer to the surface — that's why you bleed so much when you cut your lip.) In some cases, inflammation from angioedema can cause discomfort and temporary facial swelling.

>> In rare cases, angioedema can cause life-threatening swelling of the tongue, throat, and airways.

>> Angioedema often coexists with hives, but the two conditions can also occur independently. Among adults, angioedema develops in almost half of all hives cases in the United States. In approximately 40 percent of adult cases of hives, angioedema isn't present. Angioedema that occurs alone (without hives) accounts for only 10 percent of adult cases. However, these types of cases often cause doctors special concern because angioedema that occurs alone can indicate a serious underlying disorder, such as hereditary angioedema (HAE), or it can indicate a severe drug reaction.

Determining the Nature of Your Skin Condition

Hives and angioedema can erupt as a result of different allergic and nonallergic mechanisms, including various irritants, allergens, underlying medical conditions, and other factors. These mechanisms provide the basis that doctors use to categorize hives and angioedema outbreaks, as we explain in the following sections.

Allergic mechanisms: Foods, drugs, and insects

Allergic mechanisms that trigger hives and angioedema are the result of systemic allergic reactions that involve IgE antibodies (see Chapter 2 for more information). The triggers usually include substances in certain foods, medications, and insect stings.

Use the following list to gather more information on the allergic substances that trigger hives and angioedema:

>> **Foods:** Peanuts, shellfish, fish, tree nuts, eggs, milk, soy, wheat, sesame, and certain fruits are the most significant sources of allergen that can trigger hives as part of an allergic reaction in sensitized individuals. Food additives, including sodium benzoate and sulfites; food dyes, such a tartrazine; and substances in some vitamin products and dietary supplements can also trigger hive eruptions. (See Chapter 14 for more information on food hypersensitivities.)

>> **Drugs:** Penicillin, sulfa drugs and other antibiotics, aspirin, NSAIDs, insulin, narcotic pain relievers, muscle relaxers, and tranquilizers can trigger hives and angioedema as part of a systemic reaction if you're sensitized to the allergens that these products contain. (See Chapter 16 for more information on drug reactions.)

>> **Insects:** Yellow jackets, honeybees, wasps, hornets, and fire ants (all members of the *Hymenoptera* order) most commonly cause allergic reactions from their stings. Aside from the pain and discomfort of unfriendly encounters with these creatures, the reaction that most sensitized people experience is a variable degree of localized swelling at the site of the sting. However, in some rare cases, *anaphylaxis* (a life-threatening reaction that affects many organs simultaneously) can follow an insect sting or bite. Chapter 17 provides you with more information on diagnosing and treating insect stings, as well as dealing with cases of anaphylactic shock.

>> **Arachnids:** The Lone Star Tick in the United States has been found to be a vector for the production of urticarial and anaphylactic reactions to red meat. The chemical responsible for this reaction is galactose, 1-3, alpha-galactose (alpha-gal) with which the tick bite sensitizes the human victim to the sugar, causing alpha-gal syndrome (AGS). Subsequent ingestion of meat such as beef or pork can cause a significant allergic response. That's now a frequent cause of reactions in large portions of the southern United States and is rapidly spreading across the country.

Arachnids aren't insects. They have different physical characteristics and anatomies that distinguish them from each other. Insects have six legs, wings and antennae, while arachnids have eight legs and no antennae or wings. Arachnids include spiders, ticks, mites, and scorpions while insects include ants, bees, wasps, and flies. We suggest avoiding both groups whenever possible.

Physical mechanisms

Exposure to certain types of light, cold, heat, pressure, and exercise can also trigger reactions that cause hives and angioedema. Physicians refer to this type of skin condition, which accounts for nearly 20 percent of hives and angioedema cases, as *physical urticaria* or chronic inducible urticaria. Under certain circumstances — depending on factors such as your occupation, activities, and sensitivity to triggering mechanisms — you can experience various manifestations of physical urticaria simultaneously, because different forms can coexist. The most common mechanisms of chronic inducible urticaria that have been identified include the following:

» **Dermatographism:** The ability to write letters or other symbols by stroking your skin with your fingernails or a retracted ballpoint pen, for example, which results in *blanching* (whitening of your skin) that's followed by redness and swelling, is the most obvious sign of this almost harmless form of hives (some doctors also refer to this condition as *urticaria factita*). Dermatographism affects approximately 5 percent of the U.S. population and can persist for years until the outbreaks disappear. Common triggers for dermatographism include rubbing, scratching, or stroking the skin. Tight clothing or pressure from leaning against hard surfaces (a chair or desk) can also cause this form of hives. A rarer, more severe form of dermatographism — known as *symptomatic dermatographism* — can occur following bacterial, fungal, or scabies infections, or after treating a bacterial infection with penicillin.

The name of this skin condition means "skin writing" in Greek (*derma* is "skin," *graphe* is "writing").

» **Cholinergic urticaria (CU):** This form of heat-induced hives (also known as *generalized heat urticaria*) causes at least 5 percent of chronic urticaria cases. In most cases, an increase in your body temperature triggers the eruption. CU is especially common among teenagers and young adults. Factors that can cause this condition include hot baths or showers, exercise, perspiration, stress, and strongly seasoned foods. The onset of CU symptoms is generally rapid, occurring within two minutes to half an hour of the triggering event. If you suffer from CU, you may experience very itchy skin, tiny hives, tingling, an elevation of body temperature, or a burning sensation before a rash appears.

>> **Cold urticaria:** In most cases of cold urticaria, symptoms develop at the site that comes into contact with a cold substance, and hives usually develop when the area reheats after removal of the cold substance. Ice cubes typically trigger this condition. Likewise, cold drinks may cause swelling of the lips and mouth. Cold urticaria can cause life-threatening reactions in cases of sudden, total-body immersion in cold water (if you fall into a half-frozen pond, for example). If you have a history of cold urticaria, your physician may warn you to stay away from all water sports that may immerse you in cold water.

>> **Delayed pressure urticaria (DPU):** As the name implies, this disorder takes time to develop; on average, from three to five hours after a triggering form of physical pressure occurs. Types of physical pressure that can trigger an attack include contact with hard surfaces, wearing tight clothes, or applauding (no, that doesn't mean you should boo — just clap gently). Likewise, the pressure from shoulder straps of handbags, backpacks, shoulder bags, and other forms of baggage can also trigger DPU.

>> **Papular urticaria:** The characteristic signs of this disorder include small groups of itchy pimples (*papules* in Latin) that often result from insect bites. This type of hives tends to affect the lower extremities more than other parts of the body. Papular urticaria symptoms often persist longer than other forms of hives, too. However, this condition doesn't involve the type of systemic reaction that can result from *Hymenoptera* insect stings. (See the preceding section for more information on the systemic reaction to *Hymenoptera* insect stings.)

>> **Vibratory angioedema (VAE):** This rare skin condition manifests as an occupational disorder, with severe itching and swelling within minutes of vibratory exposure. Common triggers include vibrations from working in industries and professions such as metal grinding, carpentry, machine and tool making, and secretarial work. Rare cases can also occur from towel rubbing, riding on motorcycles, lawn mowing, bowling, applauding, and walking. Symptoms of VAE develop within minutes of vibratory activity and affect the body surface that experiences the vibrations most intensely.

>> **Solar urticaria:** Ultraviolet (UV) light can trigger hives in some sun-sensitive people within minutes of exposure, causing solar urticaria. Characteristic symptoms include itching, swelling, and hives at the site that receives direct exposure to UV rays. Symptoms may persist from 15 minutes to three hours. When large areas of the body are exposed, systemic reactions can occur, which include coughing, wheezing, shortness of breath, and even a drop in blood pressure.

>> **Aquagenic urticaria:** The pinpoint hives characteristic of this condition usually results from skin contact with water (cold drinks, however, don't induce this condition — see the earlier bullet about cold urticaria). The hives from this condition develop around the contact site, are often very itchy, and usually fade within 15 to 90 minutes. This diagnosis should only be made in cases where an individual has a rare positive response to a water-challenge test (hives appear within 2 to 30 minutes after water is applied to the skin) and after all other possible forms of physical urticaria have been eliminated.

Exercise-induced anaphylaxis (EIA)

As its name suggests, *exercise-induced anaphylaxis (EIA)* is an anaphylactic disorder. Anaphylaxis can result from severe allergic reactions, especially due to food, drug, and insect venom triggers. (For more anaphylaxis information, see Chapter 1.)

The trigger factor of EIA is physical activity. Symptoms of this rare syndrome can develop within 2 to 30 minutes of beginning exercise and usually progress in the following stages:

>> Rash, fatigue, and an increase in body temperature.

>> Eruption of hives and angioedema.

>> Wheeziness and other respiratory difficulties, as well as nausea, diarrhea, or dizziness.

>> Severe headache, fatigue, and elevated body temperature. In most cases, all of these symptoms cease within three hours, although your headache can persist for one to two days after the onset of the condition.

As we explain in the previous section, exercise can also trigger CU. However, unlike CU, a hot bath or shower or perspiration doesn't cause EIA in the absence of exercise. Hives associated with EIA are also usually larger than those that erupt as a result of CU. Exercising in hot, humid weather and having a family history of allergies both increase the risk of EIA. Many different types of foods have been shown to cause food-dependent exercise-induced anaphylaxis (FDEIA) including wheat, shellfish, nuts, and alcohol. In these individuals exercise or food alone don't cause anaphylaxis, but only in combination do these reactions occur. In some cases, food allergies from eating specific foods too soon after exercise, may also play a significant role in triggering anaphylaxis.

If you have any symptoms of EIA, stop exercising immediately and rest. If you are concerned that this reaction is serious, then administer epinephrine and call 911.

Your physician may obtain blood work to measure *serum tryptase*, which is released in the body during anaphylaxis. This should be measured in the blood as soon as possible and up to 6 hours after the reaction to confirm that anaphylaxis has actually occurred.

Contact mechanisms

Skin contact with certain irritants and allergens can also trigger hives. The two main categories of these types of hives include

>> **Allergic contact urticaria:** Hives may erupt after handling foods such as nuts, fish, shellfish, raw potatoes, and liver. Hives may also result from contact with allergens in antibiotics, epoxy, and treated woods. Contact with latex (in rubber gloves, for instance) may also induce this form of hives, as well as formaldehyde in clothing. (See Chapter 12 for more details on latex and other contact allergens.) Hive eruptions that occur from contact with latex, formaldehyde in new clothing, and handling certain foods result from the direct contact between your skin and allergens in these products. Hives eruptions from direct, topical contact with allergens are more limited than the systemic allergic reactions that you see after ingesting food and drugs, which are more characteristic of widespread hives.

>> **Nonallergic contact urticaria:** This disorder affects people who aren't sensitized to an allergen, but who react soon after skin contact with irritants such as insect and spider hairs (not stings or bites), alcohol, sodium benzoate, acetic acid, sorbic acid, balsam of Peru, and cobalt chloride.

Intolerance reactions

WARNING

If you have an intolerance — rather than an allergy — to aspirin, NSAIDs, and other anti-inflammatory drugs, antibiotics, narcotic pain relievers, or any medications containing tartrazine (a substance in food dyes), using these products can lead to nonallergic reactions that can trigger eruptions of hives and angioedema. (We explain the difference between an allergic drug response and drug intolerance in Chapter 16.)

Urticarial vasculitis and other systemic conditions

Hereditary factors, such as a genetic predisposition to hives and angioedema, or other medical conditions, including serum sickness (potentially as a result of a delayed adverse reaction to medication — see Chapter 16) or pregnancy, can also cause eruptions. In other instances, hives can erupt as symptoms of a serious underlying disease, similar to the distinctive skin rashes that are characteristic of chicken pox and measles.

REMEMBER

The most significant forms of hives and/or angioedema related to systemic conditions include

SEE YOUR DOCTOR

>> **Pruritic urticarial papules and plaques of pregnancy (PUPPP):** This form of intensely itchy hives sometimes affects women in the third trimester of their first pregnancy. In many cases, PUPPP disappears after delivery and doesn't recur with subsequent pregnancies. Refer to Dr. Berger's book *Asthma For Dummies* (John Wiley & Sons, Inc.) for further information on medications that your physician may advise for this condition.

>> **Urticarial pigmentosa:** Pigmented lesions that swell when stroked into a cobblestone or leopard skin pattern of hives represent the characteristic sign of this rare disorder. The onset of this condition usually occurs before the age of 3 years. Because urticaria pigmentosa can serve as a warning symptom for *systemic mastocytosis* — a serious disease that can affect the bones, liver, lymph nodes, and spleen — you need to make sure that your physician examines this type of outbreak. In addition, this form of hives can complicate symptoms of other allergies, especially those involving insect stings and bites, potentially causing severe or anaphylactic reactions.

>> **Urticarial vasculitis:** The hives that can erupt as a result of this syndrome, which affects women more than men, can resemble those that result from systemic reactions to food, drug, and insect allergies. Distinguishing symptoms of this disorder include burning or painful sensations, itchy lesions, darkened skin coloring that remains even after lesions clear, and the persistence of individual outbreaks that last longer than 24 hours and can move to a new site within minutes leaving a blue bruising residual lesion after the initial hive resolves. Often a biopsy of the lesion helps to make the diagnosis. These symptoms may also indicate a more serious underlying condition such as hepatitis, mononucleosis, thyroid disorder, or rheumatoid arthritis. In the next section we explain the tests that your doctor may perform if you appear to have this form of hives.

>> **Hereditary angioedema (HAE):** The hallmark of this disorder is hives and angioedema episodes that can affect any part of your body and that aren't associated with hives. Some cases of HAE can cause swelling of the gastrointestinal (GI) tract, leading to stomach cramps, nausea, vomiting, and intestinal and abdominal pain that many resemble appendicitis symptoms and last one to two days. The most severe complication is *laryngeal edema* (throat swelling), which can potentially be fatal. You should closely monitor this symptom

because severe laryngeal obstruction can require a tracheotomy to prevent death by asphyxiation.

Treatment of HAE is directed by administering preventive replacement therapy with medications such as C1 esterase inhibitors (Cinryze, Haegarda), berotralstat (Orladeyo), or lanadelumab-flyo (Takhzyro). Acute attacks can be treated with C1 esterase inhibitor [recombinant] (Ruconest), C1-INH replacement therapy (Berinert), ecallantide (Kalbitor), or icatibant injection (Firazyr). As a result of these recently approved medications, patients and their physicians now have several options for developing an individually tailored treatment plan.

Diagnosing Hives and Angioedema

The first step in diagnosing your skin outbreak is to determine what specific condition is affecting you. As we explain in this chapter, many different allergen, irritants, physical triggers, intolerance reaction, or underlying conditions can cause your hives and angioedema.

SEE YOUR DOCTOR

In order to narrow the range of possible causes of your hives and angioedema, your physician should thoroughly evaluate your medical history and perform a complete medical exam.

Even if they can't make a precise diagnosis, your medical history and physical exam enable them to isolate the most likely causes of your eruptions, as well as to advise effective avoidance and treatment measures for your condition. Depending on the severity and extent of your outbreak, they may also refer you to a dermatologist or allergist for further consultation.

Dealing with emergency situations

WARNING

If you notice hoarseness, tongue swelling, and difficulty swallowing (symptoms typical of laryngeal edema) along with an outbreak of hives, seek immediate emergency treatment. These symptoms may represent a severe anaphylactic reaction such as EIA or a severe form of HAE. Don't waste time trying to figure out what may be causing a reaction — use your epinephrine and get to the emergency room!

After you're out of danger, you can proceed with any further needed investigation to try to get a diagnosis so you can possibly prevent similar occurrences in the future.

Taking your hives seriously

When taking your medical history, your physician should focus on the events and possible triggers in your life that might have been affecting you at the time of your outbreaks. Prepare to give them as much information as possible about items and situations such as the following:

>> Any medications (prescription or OTC products), supplements, or herbal products you take.

>> Any exposure you may have to allergens — especially food, drug, and insect stings — in your occupation, school, home, or outdoors.

>> Any exposure to physical urticaria triggers, including cold, heat, pressure, vibrations, sunlight, and other factors that we explain in the section "Physical mechanisms" earlier in this chapter.

>> Viral or bacterial infections that you've recently experienced, including upper respiratory ailments, hepatitis, infectious mononucleosis, viral herpes, or other disorders.

>> Any autoimmune disorder such as rheumatoid arthritis or lupus erythematous.

>> Any contact you may have with allergens or irritants that trigger contact urticaria. (See the section "Contact mechanisms" earlier in this chapter.)

>> If your outbreak isn't present at the time of your visit, prepare to tell your physician where the condition typically appears on your body, how many eruptions occur, how long they persist, and how often they recur. If you have a picture of your rash, make sure to share it with your physician.

Examining eruptions

In addition to closely examining your skin, your physician should also perform a general physical examination to investigate other possible underlying disorders that may be contributing to your hives and angioedema.

TECHNICAL STUFF

Other disorders that may cause itching, inflammation, or lesions resembling hives and angioedema include

>> Pregnancy; kidney, liver thyroid, and lymph disorders; and diabetes can produce chronic itching, which you may mistake as a symptom of hives.

>> Contact dermatitis (see Chapter 12), other skin disorders, skin infections (such as cellulitis), lymphedema, and injury can cause skin swelling that resembles angioedema.

>> Stevens-Johnson syndrome, a potentially serious disorder, can cause lesions that resemble hives. Patients with this syndrome typically also experience fever, burning sensations, sore throat, and general malaise.

>> Viral herpes can trigger lesions that resemble outbreaks of papular and/ or cholinergic urticaria. If your lesions appear in a symmetrical pattern, however, you may suffer from viral herpes.

>> Serum sickness may trigger eruptions and other symptoms similar to the anaphylactic reaction of drug and insect allergies. With serum sickness, though, joint pain and fever also accompany the eruptions, and the reaction usually progresses more slowly than allergic cases.

TIP

If you're not sure whether your eruptions are hives, and if your outbreaks are infrequent and subside before you can see a physician, take color photographs (not black and white) of your eruptions with your smartphone while you can still see them. Showing these pictures to your physician can help in making a diagnosis in some cases.

Keeping a diet diary

SEE YOUR DOCTOR

In cases of intermittent eruptions that may be due to food allergies, your physician may advise you to keep track of what you consume. You usually need to record the foods and liquids that you ingest 24 hours before each episode of hives. Using this process can help you and your physician possibly pinpoint potential food-related triggers of your condition.

WARNING

Make sure that you consult with your physician before assuming that you've identified a food allergen that triggers your hives and angioedema. Arbitrarily restricting your diet or the diet of a child who suffers from hives because of a suspected food allergy can cause nutritional deficiencies.

Testing for hives

Depending on what your physician suspects as the trigger of your hives and angioedema, they may recommend certain medical tests to more precisely determine the causes and mechanisms of your condition. These tests may include the following types of procedures:

>> **Challenge tests:** If a form of physical urticaria seems the likely cause of your condition, your physician may perform procedures that provoke a small-scale reaction, similar to your outbreak. In most cases, these tests involve exposing your skin to a suspected physical mechanism such as heat, cold, UV light, pressure, water, or vibrations. Testing for exercise-induced anaphylaxis may

involve eating and then exercising in a controlled setting to determine more precisely what combination of factors may trigger an anaphylactic reaction.

>> **Allergy skin tests:** Your physician may find skin testing for allergens useful when evaluating the cause of acute urticaria. In contrast with CSU, allergies more often cause eruptions in acute cases. (For more information on allergy skin testing, see Chapter 4.)

>> **Blood tests:** If allergy skin testing is not advisable, your doctor may recommend an ImmunoCAP blood test (see Chapter 4).

>> **Skin punch biopsy:** This test involves extracting a small skin sample from your affected area for laboratory analysis. Doctors usually only perform a skin punch biopsy if they suspect that urticarial vasculitis causes your hives and if other lab tests show inconclusive results. A dermatologist usually performs the procedure, and a pathologist, who specializes in reading skin biopsies, evaluates the results.

Managing Hives: I Can't Go Out Like This

Avoidance measures and symptom relief are the keys to effective management of hives and angioedema. Some hives and angioedema cases resolve without major medical intervention and only require simple self-care and occasional medication to manage eruptions and associated symptoms (especially itching). Likewise, if you experience occasional outbreaks, you can improve your condition without treatment so long as you avoid exposure to the substances or mechanisms that trigger your symptoms.

If the cause of your eruptions is difficult to determine or if your outbreaks are more serious and persistent, your physician may prescribe a preventive course of medication to help keep your condition from adversely affecting your quality of life. In the event of a widespread outbreak, seek immediate emergency medical attention.

Relieving the hives on your own

In addition to avoiding allergens, irritants, mechanisms, and intolerance reactions that may trigger your hives and angioedema, the most important concept to keep in mind when dealing with outbreaks is not to make your condition worse.

TIP

If an outbreak occurs, follow these recommendations to relieve your symptoms and avoid making them worse:

>> **Bathe and wash with lukewarm water.** Avoid hot baths and showers because they may intensify your symptoms and may also trigger conditions such as cholinergic urticaria. Likewise, avoid cold water and handling frozen items — such as ice cubes — because they can trigger cold urticaria outbreaks. (See the section "Physical mechanisms" earlier in this chapter.)

>> **Don't use harsh soaps.** Using harsh soaps can damage your skin's natural protective layer and cause more itchiness. The less you itch, the less likely you're to infect your lesions through scratching.

>> **Apply moisturizers immediately after bathing and avoid brisk drying.** Instead, gently use a soft towel to pat yourself dry.

>> **Sport the loose look.** Wear comfortable, cotton, lightweight clothes, and avoid tight, restrictive garments.

>> **Stay out of hot environments as much as possible at work, home, or school.** Try to keep your home cool, especially your bedroom.

WARNING

>> **Avoid using any type of aspirin or NSAIDs, even after your outbreaks subside.** If you need medication for everyday aches and pains, your doctor may advise you to use acetaminophen products such as Tylenol. Likewise, avoid using alcohol or narcotic pain relievers.

Relying on medication

Physicians mainly prescribe antihistamines from the H-1 class (see the nearby sidebar) to relieve and prevent the symptoms that accompany hives and angioedema. However, your physician may prescribe more potent drugs if you suffer from more severe or persistent outbreaks. We discuss both types here.

Oral antihistamines

Antihistamines block the inflammatory effects of histamine to help reduce inflammation and can often relieve the itching associated with outbreaks of hives and angioedema. Your physician may prescribe a less-sedating (Zyrtec) or a nonsedating second-generation H-1 antihistamine (Allegra, Claritin). In patients with uncontrolled urticaria who are treated with second-generation antihistamines, a 4-fold higher dose can be used until symptoms are controlled. Your physician may then consider *step-down dosing* (meaning that they may recommend stepping down your level of medication if you've been able to consistently achieve good control of your symptoms).

Your physician may prescribe an OTC-sedating antihistamine such as Benadryl if you can't sleep at night because of the discomfort from inflammation and itching. If these products don't provide you with sufficient relief, your physician may prescribe a combination of an H-1 with an H-2 class antihistamine such as Pepcid. (See the nearby sidebar for more information on H-1 and H-2 antihistamines.)

Other medications

If H-1 and H-2 antihistamine combinations fail to provide sufficient symptom relief, your physician may consider prescribing more potent drugs. These drugs can include the following:

>> **Prescription first-generation antihistamines:** These drugs can effectively treat cases of chronic hives that don't respond to prescription second-generation H-1 antihistamines. In some cases, your physician may also prescribe a combination of prescription first-generation antihistamines with products from other antihistamine classes. For example, physicians often prescribe hydroxyzine (Atarax) to treat cases of CU and as a preventive treatment for dermatographism. Cyproheptadine (Periactin) achieves good results in treating cold urticaria. However, because these products have sedating side effects that can significantly interfere with your daily life, your physician may advise that you only use these drugs at night.

>> **Antidepressants:** Doxepin (Sinequan) often provides a powerful antihistamine effect that your physician may use to treat chronic hives. As with hydroxyzine and cyproheptadine, doxepin causes sedation, which may limit its use in some cases.

>> **Biologics:** Omalizumab (Xolair) is approved for treatment of CSU in patient 6 years and older and is given by injection starting at a dose of 300 mg every four weeks. If there's an insufficient response, the dose can be increased to a maximum of 600mg every two weeks. The patient should be allowed up to 6 months to achieve a response. The addition of omalizumab has revolutionized the treatment of hives because it has been greatly effective in most patients while being extremely safe.

>> **Immunosuppressants:** Cyclosporine is a medication that works by suppressing immune system responses. It can be of therapeutic value in patients with CSU that is unresponsive to conventional therapy. However, it can reduce your ability to fight off infections and can cause high blood pressure and kidney problems. The risk of these problems increases with higher doses and prolonged treatment with this drug.

>> **Corticosteroids:** If your hives and angioedema are particularly severe, extensive, and persistent, your physician may prescribe a short course of oral corticosteroids, such as prednisone. If prednisone doesn't prove effective, they may instead prescribe methylprednisolone (Medrol). Likewise, if your

condition relapses after one of two short courses of these medications, they may decide, as a last resort, to prescribe alternate-day single morning oral corticosteroid therapy for several weeks. If they decide that you need this therapy, you must remain under close medical supervision for the duration of the medication course and make sure that you don't miss any of your scheduled appointments with your physician. You should also make sure that they provide clearly written instructions for your dosage schedule before you leave the office. Unfortunately, corticosteroids can cause serious side effects with long-term use. Therefore, they should best be administered in short doses of a few days, no more than three times a year.

TIP

>> **Oral antibiotics and antihistamines:** In case where bacterial infection develops — usually from scratching itchy rashes and lesions — we recommend using oral antihistamines to relieve itching and oral antibiotics to clear your infection. Using topical forms of these medications can result in allergic sensitization to these drugs, so you should clearly avoid topical forms when treating inflamed skin.

WARNING

>> **Emergency medication:** In the event that you suffer from a severe angioedema outbreak or an anaphylactic reaction that causes your tongue and mouth to swell and interfere with your breathing, you may need an emergency injection of epinephrine (EpiPen, Auvi-Q), or the newly approved epinephrine nasal spray (neffy) as the initial treatment for anaphylaxis, to help keep your airway open and reduce swelling. (See Chapter 1 for information on dealing with anaphylaxis.)

CLASSIFYING ANTIHISTAMINES

Antihistamines are classified by the types of histamine receptors, H-1 or H-2, that the drugs are designed to block. Your nasal cells have H-1 receptors, and your gastric (stomach) cells have H-2 receptors. Most people associate H-1 antihistamines with the treatment of allergies. However, your skin possesses both types of receptors, and your allergies may therefore require treatment with both H-1 and H-2 antihistamines.

Although the H-2 receptors in your stomach cells release histamine that secretes heartburn-causing acid, the release of histamine from H-2 receptors in your skin's blood vessels may also cause itching, swelling, and the development of hives. Therefore, H-2 antihistamines, such as famotidine (Pepcid), which is primarily marketed for relief of peptic ulcers and heartburn, can, in combination with H-1 antihistamines, provide a more comprehensive treatment of itching, swelling, and hives. Although these medications are generally safe, you should only use these products for the relief of hives and angioedema (or other medical conditions) on the advice of your physician.

5
Reviewing Food, Drug, and Insect Allergies

Chapter **14**

Diagnosing and Managing Food Allergies

I f the food you eat bites you back with outbreaks of eczema, gastric distress, fits of wheezing, or other symptoms (perhaps even including life-threatening bouts of anaphylactic shock), you're not alone. Adverse food reactions affect at least one in four Americans at some point in their lives.

REMEMBER

However, not all food ingredients that can cause adverse reactions are triggers of *food hypersensitivity* (the more precise term for *food allergy*). Even through 40 percent of Americans believe that their unfortunate gastronomical experiences result from allergies to certain foods, most cases involve various forms of food intolerance, food poisoning, and other nonallergic conditions we explain throughout this chapter.

In fact, although allergic reactions to food can be severe (and should be appropriately diagnosed and managed), the actual number of adults in the United States who suffer from food hypersensitivities is significantly lower than 40 percent. That being said, true IgE mediated food allergy has been increasing steadily over the last two decades and is now estimated to affect 4 to 8 percent of children and up to 10 percent of adults.

Distinguishing between Food Hypersensitivity and Intolerance

Because the range of adverse food reactions can include a constellation of nasal, respiratory, skin, gastrointestinal, and oral symptoms occurring separately or in combination, physicians usually classify these reactions according to the mechanisms that the reactions involve.

REMEMBER

The following list provides a summary of the two main classifications of adverse food reactions:

>> **Food hypersensitivity:** These reactions occur when your immune system responds to specific proteins in certain food. The reactions can include allergic mechanisms involving IgE antibodies (see Chapter 1) as well as nonallergic mechanisms, which we explain in the next two sections of this chapter.

- Allergic food hypersensitivities include gastrointestinal (GI) tract allergies, hives and other allergic skin reactions, and even *anaphylaxis* (a severe, abrupt reaction that affects many organs of the body simultaneously and can potentially be life-threatening).

- Nonallergic food hypersensitivities (sometimes referred to as *non- IgE food reactions*) include syndromes such as food protein-induced enterocolitis syndrome (FPIES), colitis, and malabsorption, as well as celiac disease, dermatitis herpetiformis, and pulmonary hypersensitivity. We discuss these medical conditions in greater detail in "Understanding Nonallergic (Non-IgE) Food hypersensitivities," later in this chapter.

>> **Food intolerance:** These types of reactions result from nonallergic, nonimmunologic responses to offending substances in various foods. Forms of food intolerance include

- Lactose intolerance

- Pharmacologic food reactions

- Metabolic food reactions

- Food additive reactions

- Food poisoning

- Toxic reactions

Identifying Different Types of Food Hypersensitivities

In the case of an *IgE-meditated food hypersensitivity*, commonly known as a *food allergy*, your immune system cooks up specific IgE antibodies (see Chapter 1) against specific allergens. The level of exposure required for your immune system to be sensitized to a particular food varies, depending on the allergens involved.

Recognizing the common food culprits

Although most people's diets typically include hundreds of different foods, it turns out that only nine foods are responsible for more than 90 percent of the food allergy reactions. The major food allergens that have been identified are mostly proteins often found in the following foods and are listed here in the order of how commonly they occur:

>> Peanuts (the leading cause of severe allergic food reactions), soybeans, peas, lentils, beans and other legumes, and foods containing these products as ingredients. Because a wide variety of foods include peanuts and soybean products as ingredients, these legumes often act as hidden triggers of food allergies. In the section "Anaphylaxis and allergic food reactions," later in this chapter, we provide more information on peanut issues. You can find details on uncovering hidden allergenic ingredients in many common foods in Chapter 15.

>> Shellfish, including crustaceans and mollusks, such as shrimp, lobster, crab, mussels, clams, and oysters, accounts for 2.9 percent of food allergy.

>> Cow's milk and products that contain milk protein fractions, such as casein (80 percent of the protein in cow's milk) and whey, which includes lactalbumin and lactoglobulin. Cow's milk allergy affects approximately 2 percent of the population.

>> Finned fish — both freshwater and saltwater — has been reported to affect 0.9 percent of the population.

>> Tree nuts, including almonds, Brazil nuts, cashews, hazelnuts, and walnuts. Tree nut allergy prevalence is estimated to be 1.2 percent of the population.

>> Eggs, especially egg whites, which contain the predominant allergenic proteins, ovalbumin, and ovomucoid. The yolk is considered less allergenic that the egg white. Egg allergy is more common in young children who tend to grow out of their allergy as they age. However, it can persist in some people who are severely allergic to eggs. Overall, the estimated incidence of egg allergy is less than 1 percent of the population.

>> Wheat, an important ingredient in bran, malt, wheat flour, graham flour, wheat germ, and wheat starch. Corn, rice, barley, oats, and other grains and cereals are less common food allergy triggers. Not to be confused with celiac disease, (which is a sensitivity to a component of gluten in wheat), true wheat allergy is considerably less common, affecting less then 1 percent of the population.

>> Sesame is a common ingredient in many foods, including baked goods and savory dishes. As recently as January 2023, sesame was added to the major list of allergens that are required to be labeled on all commercially packaged foods, as part of the revised labeling laws. This is due to its increasing prevalence in the United States where sesame allergy has been reported in 0.8 percent of the population.

>> Soy is commonly used ingredient in many foods, including breads, cookies, crackers, and soups. Soybeans are particularly found in Asian cuisine such as tofu, edamame, soy sauce, soy nuts, and sprouts. Soy allergy is more common in infants and young children than in older kids, affecting approximately 0.4 percent of infants in the United States.

Both the prevalence and type of food allergies often differ between adults and children. For example, of these common ingested culprits, the products that trigger allergic food reactions in children most frequently are milk, eggs, peanuts, tree nuts, fish, soy, and wheat. In adults, the likeliest causes of allergic food reactions include fish, shellfish, peanuts, and tree nuts.

Although most children lose their sensitivity to milk and eggs by age 3, food allergies involving peanuts, fish shellfish, and tree nuts tend to persist and may last a lifetime.

Other, less-obvious sources of food allergens may possibly cause adverse reactions in a smaller number of susceptible individuals. These much less-frequently problematic food allergens (listed in family groupings to keep it all in the family) include the following:

>> **Lily family:** Onions, leeks, garlic, asparagus

>> **Mustard family:** Broccoli, cabbage, cauliflower, horseradish, turnip, radish, mustard

>> **Plum family:** Apricots, cherries, peaches, almonds, plums

>> **Gourd family:** Watermelon, honeydew, cantaloupe, other melons, pumpkins, squash

>> **Nightshade family:** Tomatoes, potatoes, eggplant, bell pepper, red pepper

ADDITIVES AND ALLERGIES

Allergic mechanisms may or may not play a part in some adverse food reactions commonly associated with food additives. When additives are in the picture, identifying a suspected food allergen can get complicated because finding out whether the food itself or the additive causes the problem is often difficult.

Additives such as sulfites are often used as antioxidants to preserve wine, dried fruit, shrimp, and potatoes. These additives have been implicated in cases of allergic food hypersensitivities, including potentially life-threatening *bronchospasm* (constriction of the airways) and asthma symptoms, especially in severe asthmatics who require long-term treatment with oral corticosteroids.

Exposure to sulfites, when used in salad bars and in the guacamole served in some restaurants, can trigger asthma symptoms in susceptible asthmatics when they inhale the sulfite fumes from treated foods. These antioxidant additives are sometimes used to prevent discoloration and to keep greens looking pretty. That's why some salad bar lettuce — which may sit out for hours during the day — doesn't seem to wilt, unlike the salads most people prepare at home.

The U.S. Food and Drug Administration (FDA) prohibits using sulfites on fresh fruits and vegetables meant to be eaten raw (as with a salad bar) and requires manufacturers to label products that contain sulfites. However, pre-cut or peeled potato products used in some restaurants to make common side dishes (such as french fries and hash browns) may still contain sulfites. Therefore, if you have asthma, we advise always asking questions about the food served in restaurants.

Physicians often need to be detectives to determine the cause of adverse food reactions. For example, if you experience an adverse food reaction to a hot dog, your physician must determine whether your reaction is because of allergens in the meat, whether you're suffering from hot dog headache due to nitrites used to retard meat spoilage, or whether you're reacting to added food dye that creates the pink color.

How allergic food hypersensitivities develop

Atopy, the genetic predisposition to develop allergies, is a significant factor in the development of food hypersensitivity. An infant's immune system can begin responding to food allergies soon after birth.

As we explain in Chapter 1, your inherited tendency to develop allergies can express itself in other allergic conditions also, such as allergic rhinitis (hay fever) and atopic dermatitis (eczema). Your allergies may progress and evolve over time. This process is known as the *atopic march*. The predisposition toward allergies passes between generations, but the specific allergies themselves may not. Therefore, Mom may be allergic to lobster, Junior may break out in hives after eating peanuts, and baby Betty may get congested after drinking cow's milk formula.

The severity of your symptoms may also depend on the level of your sensitivity to particular food allergens and the quantities of these foods you consume. In some cases, ingesting small amounts of these foods may not trigger adverse reactions. The following section provides more detail on the various forms of allergic food hypersensitivities.

Gastrointestinal tract allergies

Allergic reactions involving the digestive system can develop within a few minutes to several hours after ingesting food allergens, and they frequently result in abdominal pain, vomiting, and diarrhea. The most significant classifications of gastrointestinal (GI) allergies include

>> **Gastrointestinal food hypersensitivity reaction:** This reaction generally occurs with other atopic conditions, such as allergic rhinitis and atopic dermatitis, and can cause nausea, stomach pain, vomiting, and, in some cases, diarrhea. In rare cases, a widespread systemic reaction such as anaphylaxis can also result. (See the section "Anaphylaxis and allergic food reactions" later in this chapter.)

>> **Cow's milk allergy:** Approximately 2 to 3 percent of infants develop allergies to the proteins in casein and whey (including lactalbumin and lactoglobulin) in cow's milk, resulting in adverse reactions (such as colic, vomiting, and diarrhea) even to minute amounts of these proteins. This reaction isn't the same as the more familiar syndrome know as *lactose intolerance*, as we explain in the section "Focusing On Food Intolerance" later in this chapter.

>> **Allergic eosinophilic gastroenteropathy:** This rare condition can cause nausea and vomiting following meals, abdominal pain, and diarrhea. If not managed effectively, this type of allergy can result in malabsorption and malnutrition, leading potentially to stunted or slowed growth in infants and weight loss in adults.

>> **Alpha-Gal syndrome:** This type of food allergy occurs when people are allergic to red meat and other products derived from mammals. This syndrome usually starts with the bite of the Lone Star tick, mainly in the southern parts of the United States. The tick bite transfers a sugar molecule, which is a carbohydrate called *alpha-gal* into the body, causing the body's immune system to respond. The only treatment requires avoiding red meat and

averting tick bites by wearing long pants and long-sleeved shirts when in wooded areas.

>> **Oral allergy syndrome (OAS) or pollen food allergy syndrome (PFAS):** If you have allergic rhinitis (hay fever), you also experience oral allergy symptoms after consuming certain fresh fruits and raw vegetables. This cross-reactivity syndrome can occur if you're sensitive to ragweed pollen (with bananas and melons such as cantaloupe, honeydew, and watermelon), birch pollen (with apples, carrots, potatoes, hazelnuts, and members of the plum family), and mugwort pollen (with celery, apple, and kiwi fruit). Your symptoms may include severe itching and swelling of the lips, tongue, and palate, as well as blistering of the throat and mucus lining of the mouth. You may be able to consume these fruits and vegetables in cooked or frozen forms; they seem to trigger reactions only in their raw state. However, make sure that you check with your physician before you cook up that vegetable stir-fry or cool off with a melon sorbet.

Hives and other food-related skin reactions

Allergic food hypersensitivities involving the IgE antibodies can also trigger skin reactions in people whose atopic predisposition shows up through skin conditions. These conditions include

>> **Atopic dermatitis (eczema):** In more than one-third of children affected by this skin condition, eggs, milk, peanuts, tree nuts, soybean, and wheat can contribute to outbreaks. (See Chapter 11 for more details on atopic dermatitis.)

>> **Urticaria (hives):** These itchy welts can erupt from various types of reactions to many foods including peanuts, tree nuts, milk, eggs, fish, shellfish, soybeans, and fruits; as well as food additives such as sodium benzoates, sulfites, and food dyes. Skin contact with raw meats, fish, vegetables, and fruit can also trigger eruptions of acute contact urticaria. Allergic-food hypersensitivities are more likely to act as triggers of *rapid onset urticaria* (a particularly quick and severe eruption of hives) in children than in adults. (See Chapter 13 for more information on hives.) Food-related exercise-induced anaphylaxis (EIA), which we discuss in the next section, can also trigger hives and angioedema.

>> **Angioedema:** Also known as *deep swellings*, this condition results in deeper tissue inflammation, causing swelling of the skin, and is more likely to produce painful and burning sensations rather than itching. Angioedema can erupt as a reaction to the same food allergens that trigger hives (Chapter 13 provides more details on angioedema)

WARNING

In severe cases of hives and angioedema, symptoms can also include swelling of the tongue, throat, airway, and difficulty swallowing, as well as fainting. If angioedema affects your face, the swelling many potentially lead to breathing difficulties. If you experience swelling of your airway, get emergency care immediately.

Anaphylaxis and allergic food reactions

The most extreme of all allergic food symptoms is *anaphylaxis*. This abrupt, systemic allergic reaction, often caused by the same foods that trigger hives and angioedema eruptions, affects several organs simultaneously and can quickly turn life-threatening.

GENERALIZED URTICARIA (TOTAL BODY HIVES)

Generalized urticaria (widespread hives occurring simultaneously over much of your body surface area) can often be the initial symptom of impending anaphylaxis and can result in a sudden swelling (*angioedema*) of the lips, eyelids, tongue, and windpipe (*laryngeal edema*), as well as wheezing and dizziness. This particularly dangerous reaction can quickly progress to anaphylaxis, leading to shock, hypotension, *arrhythmia* (irregular heartbeat), and even cardiorespiratory arrest. In rare cases, this type of reaction can be fatal.

Common triggers of total body hives include foods such as peanuts and shellfish (in people who have extreme hypersensitivities to these foods), severe allergic reactions to medications such as penicillin and related compounds (or pseudo-allergic reactions to aspirin and/or related NSAIDs; see Chapter 16), generalized hypersensitivity to latex (see Chapter 12), and/or extreme sensitivities to stings from insects of the *Hymenoptera* class, which includes honeybees, yellow jackets, wasps, hornets, and fire ants (see Chapter 17).

FOOD-DEPENDENT EXERCISE-INDUCED ANAPHYLAXIS

Food-dependent exercise-induced anaphylaxis, a variant of exercise-induced — anaphylaxis (EIA) — which we explain in Chapter 9 — can occur when you exercise within three to four hours after eating a particular food. Two forms of this condition exist:

>> In most instances, anaphylaxis results only if you ingest particular foods, especially celery, shellfish, wheat, fruit, milk, or fish prior to exercise. If you experience this type of reaction and you can identify the specific foods that trigger you episodes, your physician may advise allergy skin testing (see Chapter 3) to confirm your sensitivity to the suspected foods.

>> In rare cases, you may develop anaphylaxis while exercising, regardless of the type of food you've consumed.

MANAGING AND PREVENTING ANAPHYLAXIS

Food hypersensitivity is a leading cause of anaphylaxis. Current estimates indicate that as many as 200 people in the United States die each year from food-induced anaphylactic reactions. The most effective long-term method for preventing food-induced anaphylactic reactions is to avoid eating foods that trigger reactions. We provide more details on avoiding food allergens and establishing a safe diet in Chapter 15.

REMEMBER

If your child suffers from food-induced anaphylaxis, notify babysitters, relatives, parents of other children, daycare workers, teachers, and other school personnel of your child's sensitivities and ask if they've been trained to administer rescue medications (epinephrine).

AVOIDING PEANUT PROBLEMS IN CHILDREN

As a parent of a peanut-allergic child, you need to pay close attention to products that might contain peanuts, because they can potentially cause life-threatening anaphylactic reactions in children (as well as adults) who are extremely allergic to this food.

REMEMBER

Here are some important points to keep in mind about peanuts and children:

>> Many foods contain peanuts as a not-so-obvious added ingredient. Therefore, you should examine all food labels for peanut ingredients and carefully select menu items when dining out with a child who is allergic to peanuts. (See Chapter 15 for more information on foods that contain peanuts.) You may want to pack your child's lunch to reduce the risk of your child unknowingly consuming foods with minute traces of peanuts in school lunches.

>> Because so many foods include peanuts as ingredients, teach your young child to avoid peanuts but also never to accept foods — particularly snacks and candy bars — from others, especially classmates, playmates, and young siblings.

REMEMBER

>> Because the peanut hypersensitivity issue has received widespread media attention, some airlines are introducing peanut-free flights. If you suffer from food hypersensitivities of any kind, however, we advise asking a lot of questions about the food on your flight, even if the airline claims that no peanuts or peanut ingredients are in the snacks or meals.

SEE YOUR
DOCTOR

>> A child who has a peanut hypersensitivity should wear a MedicAlert bracelet, especially at school. Also, ask your family physician about supplying your child's school with an emergency epinephrine kit. Make sure school personnel know how and when to administer this medication. Ask for a copy of the school's emergency training policy.

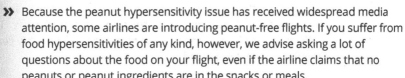

GETTING EMERGENCY TREATMENT FOR ANAPHYLAXIS

If you are prone to anaphylaxis, you should carry injectable epinephrine with you at all times and receive emergency care as soon as possible after an attack occurs.

We also advise having an emergency plan in place that includes the following items:

>> Medications your physician has prescribed for you in the event of an anaphylactic reaction

>> A list of your symptoms

>> A written treatment plan prepared by your physician

>> Your physician's name and contact information

SEE YOUR DOCTOR

Ask your physician whether an emergency epinephrine kit such as an EpiPen (or EpiPen Jr. for children under 66 pounds) or Auvi-Q, which comes in three doses: 0.3mls, 0.15ml, and 0.1mls, depending on the weight of the patient. Wear a Medi-cAlert bracelet or necklace in case you're unable to speak during a reaction.

Recently, the U.S. Food and Drug Administration approved the first non-injectable emergency treatment for allergic reactions, including life threatening anaphylaxis, in the form of a single dose epinephrine nasal spray 2 mg called "neffy."

This medication is a single dose nasal spray administered into one nostril. As with epinephrine-injection products, a second dose may be delivered, using a new nasal spray to administer neffy in the same nostril, if there is no improvement in symptoms or if symptoms worsen.

The present approval is for adult and pediatric patients who weigh at least 30 kilograms (about 66 pounds). Plans are also underway to achieve regulatory approval for a neffy 1 mg product for younger children 15 kg (33 pounds) to less than 30 kg (66 pounds) in the near future.

Neffy comes with a warning that certain nasal conditions, such as nasal polyps or a history of nasal surgery, may affect absorption of neffy. Patients with these conditions should consult with their physician and possibly consider the use of an epinephrine injector instead.

Understanding Nonallergic (Non-IgE) Food Hypersensitivities

Food hypersensitivity can also result from immune system reactions that don't involve the production of IgE antibodies. The most significant nonallergic food reactions include the following:

>> **Food protein-induced enterocolitis syndrome (FPIES):** This condition primarily occurs in infants between one and three months of age. Characteristic symptoms include prolonged vomiting and diarrhea, often resulting in dehydration. Triggers are usually the proteins in formulas that contain cow's milk or substitutes. Occasionally, breast-fed infants may also suffer from this syndrome, presumably as the result of a protein ingested by the mother and transferred to the infant in maternal milk. Similar symptoms can occur in older children and adults in response to eggs, rice, wheat, and peanuts. However, most children outgrow this type of hypersensitivity by their third birthday.

>> **Food-induced colitis:** Cow's milk and soy protein hypersensitivity have been implicated in this disorder, which can occur in the first few months of life and is usually diagnosed through the presence of blood in the stools, either seen by the naked eye or hidden (*occult*), of children who otherwise appear healthy. This condition often diminishes after six months to two years if children avoid the implicated food allergens.

TIP

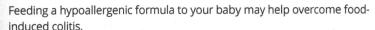

Feeding a hypoallergenic formula to your baby may help overcome food-induced colitis.

>> **Malabsorption syndrome:** This condition involves hypersensitivity to proteins in foods such as cow's milk, soy, wheat and other cereal grains and eggs. Symptoms include diarrhea, vomiting, and weight loss or failure to gain weight.

>> **Celiac disease:** This condition is a more serious form of malabsorption syndrome, and it can cause intestinal inflammation. Symptoms range from diarrhea and abdominal cramping to anemia and osteoporosis. Celiac disease only seems to occur in people who inherit an atopic predisposition. Affected individuals develop a hypersensitivity to a component of gluten called *gliadin*, which you find in wheat, rye, and barley. If you suffer from this syndrome, however, you're not necessarily doomed to a life without pasta and pancakes: Resourceful sufferers of celiac disease have come up with many gluten-free products, ranging from beer to pretzels.

>> **Dermatitis herpetiformis:** This condition is a non-IgE-mediated food hypersensitivity to gluten that produces skin eruptions in addition to causing

intestinal inflammation. Typical symptoms include a chronic itchy rash that appears primarily on the elbows, knees, and buttocks, although the disease can affect other areas as well.

>> **Pulmonary hypersensitivity:** This rare condition, induced by cow's milk, primarily affects young children. Characteristic symptoms include a chronic cough, wheezing, and severe anemia. Removing the offending dairy products from the diet can substantially alleviate symptoms.

Focusing On Food Intolerance

Many adverse food reactions don't involve an immune system response. These types of direct, non-immunologic reactions are considered signs and symptoms of food intolerance and include the conditions that we explain in the following sections.

Lactose intolerance

If you're lactose intolerant, odds are your body doesn't produce sufficient amounts of the lactase enzyme in order for you to properly digest cow's milk. If you drink milk or consume foods with high milk content, you may experience stomach cramps, bloating, nausea, gas, and diarrhea.

TIP

Avoiding cow's milk and cow's milk products or adding the lactase enzyme to those foods are the standard ways of managing lactose intolerance. In contrast with cow's-milk allergy (which we mention in the section "Identifying Different Types of Food Hypersensitivities" earlier in this chapter), you may be able to consume small quantities of cow's milk without suffering an adverse reaction.

Metabolic food reactions

In some cases, eating average or normal amounts of particular foods (especially fatty foods) may disrupt your digestive system because of various factors. These disruptions, called *metabolic food reactions*, may be caused by

>> Medications (for example, antibiotics) you're taking for illnesses

>> A disease or condition (such as gastrointestinal virus) that may affect your digestive system

>> Malnutrition (for example, due to vitamin or enzyme deficiency)

SEE YOUR DOCTOR

Consult your physician if everyday foods disrupt your digestive system frequently, especially if a prescribed medication seems to contribute to the condition.

Pharmacologic food reactions

WARNING

More serious forms of metabolic food reactions can result if you combine certain foods and drugs that don't mix well. Beware of the following potentially dangerous combinations:

SEE YOUR DOCTOR

>> Grapefruit juice, which is usually harmless, sometimes causes harmful interactions when consumed by patients taking calcium channel blockers, such as Procardia.

SEE YOUR DOCTOR

If you have a heart condition, ask your physician about possible interactions between grapefruit juice and any over-the-counter (OTC) or prescription antihistamines you may take.

>> If you take blood-thinning drugs such as Coumadin, check with your physician before eating foods rich in vitamin K such as broccoli, spinach, and turnip greens, because these foods can reduce the medications' effectiveness.

SEE YOUR DOCTOR

>> A harmful potassium buildup can occur if you overindulge in bananas while taking ACE inhibitors, such as Capoten and Vasotec.

>> Avoid foods high in tyramine, such as cheese and sausage, if you take MAO inhibitors, because the combination can cause a potentially fatal rise in blood pressure. Tyramine may also aggravate or trigger migraine headaches.

>> The caffeine in coffee, tea, and colas can interact badly with ulcer medications such as Tagamet, Zantac, and Pepcid AC. If your physician prescribes theophylline for your asthma, you should reduce your caffeine intake, because caffeine can worsen side effects of the medication such as GI irritation, headache, jitteriness, and sleeplessness.

Food additive reactions

Physicians associate many types of food additives with adverse food reactions. The most frequently implicated food additives are

>> **Monosodium glutamate (MSG):** When consumed in large quantities, this flavor enhancer causes burning sensations, facial pressure, chest pain, headache, and, in rare cases, severe asthma symptoms. Although many sufferers associate these types of reactions with eating Chinese or other types of Asian foods, no conclusive studies have determined a clear link between

consuming MSG and adverse food reactions. In any event, with the recent increase of MSG-free restaurants in many parts of the United States, you should have no trouble finding a place to chow down on chow mein without suffering ill effects.

>> **Tartrazine (yellow dye #5):** This and other food dyes can aggravate chronic hives and may actually be an ingredient in the very same children's syrups used to treat allergic symptoms such as hives — another good reason to always check medication labels.

WARNING

>> **Sulfites:** Commonly found in processed foods and almost always in wines, sulfites can produce respiratory difficulties. In rare cases, sulfites can also trigger potentially life-threatening *bronchospasm* (constriction of the airways) and asthma symptoms in some individuals (see the sidebar in this chapter about additives).

Food poisoning

WARNING

Food poisoning can result from bacterial contamination of improperly prepared or handled foods, especially meats or salads. You've probably heard of bacterial bad guys such as salmonella, *e. coli, listeria, staphylococcus enterotoxin,* and *clostridia botulinum.* These pathogenic bacteria are the usual suspects in outbreaks of food poisoning. Symptoms of food poisoning typically include nausea, vomiting, and diarrhea and can often mimic the flu. In rare cases, food-poisoning reactions can be fatal if not treated in time.

Researchers believe that many cases of illnesses mistakenly diagnosed as the 24-hour flu bug are actually the result of ingesting tainted foods.

REMEMBER

If many people develop similar symptoms after the eating the same meal, (the potato salad with especially rich mayonnaise that sat in the sun all afternoon at the family picnic, for example), food poisoning is the likely cause of all those urgent trips to the restroom.

TIP

If you experience severe gastric distress that seems related to food poisoning, make sure you drink enough liquid to avoid dehydration, which is one of the most serious adverse effects of this reaction. If your condition doesn't improve within 24 hours, seek medical attention.

Toxic food reactions

Some foods are intrinsically poisonous to all humans, regardless of allergies or other conditions. Poisonous mushrooms, such as the Amanita variety, for example, are among the most dangerous foods you can consume. Other potent sources of toxic food reactions include shellfish caught in a red tide and exotic fish such as puffers, which can cause fatal reactions when consumed unless you prepare them properly.

WARNING

Use caution when picking those pretty toadstools during your hike through the forest. In some cases, the prettier the food, the more toxic it can be. Make sure your children (and you, for that matter) don't eat toxic garden plants such as azaleas, mistletoe, rhododendrons, jimsonweed, and daffodils.

Toxic food reactions can affect both the central nervous system and digestive system, causing symptoms such as

>> Delirium, dizziness, unconsciousness, and convulsions.

>> Breathing difficulties.

>> Stomach cramps, nausea, vomiting, and diarrhea.

>> Burning or severe pain in the mouth, throat, and stomach. (These symptoms characterize poisoning that occur when you ingest poisonous products such as household or garden chemicals.)

REMEMBER

If you suspect that you or someone around you is experiencing a toxic reaction, contact your local Poison Control Center by telephone 1-800-222-1222 or https://triage.webpoisoncontrol.org/#!/exclusions. Toxic reactions very often require immediate emergency medical care.

Chapter **15**

Understanding and Treating Food Allergies

As we discuss in Chapter 14, adverse reactions to foods are common and can present in many different forms. Even though true food allergy (food hypersensitivity) accounts for only a small proportion of these negative reactions to foods, it tends to be the most severe type of adverse food reaction. In fact, food allergies are the leading cause of *anaphylaxis*, a severe allergic reaction that can become life-threatening very quickly without rapid medical intervention.

If you or your loved one has recently been diagnosed with a food allergy, or if you suspect you've developed one, feeling confused and even a little overwhelmed is perfectly normal. For example, you might even be wondering why your body is suddenly reacting to a food that never caused problems for you previously.

This chapter dives into the science behind food allergies and explains how your immune system plays a key role in this condition. We discuss the various approaches your physician uses to determine whether you have a true IgE-mediated food allergy — and its likely cause — using investigative tools such as food diaries and diagnostic tests.

Although no cure currently exists for food allergy, what if it could actually be prevented? This chapter examines new evidence, which contradicts previous guidance that recommended avoiding food allergens in early life in order to prevent the onset of food allergies. We also explore the exciting new field of food allergy treatments that extend beyond strict allergen avoidance and offers hope for the future of food allergy management as more treatment options become available.

Looking Closer at the Immunology of Food Allergy

If you've ever experienced an allergic reaction, you may be wondering what's happening in your body to produce all those distressing symptoms. In this section, we outline the immunological processes that occur during food allergy reactions and describe the various steps that are involved.

Allergic sensitization

For the immune system to develop an IgE-mediated allergic reaction to a particular food, it must first be sensitized to the offending food allergen. *Sensitization* occurs when a person who is at risk of developing a food allergy is exposed to the food for the first time, either by eating the food or through contact with the skin.

Usually, no allergic reaction occurs at this initial stage, and so the person may be completely unaware of their impending allergic sensitization. However, a lot is happening at an immunological level at this point, as the immune system has mistakenly identified the harmless food protein as a potential threat.

The immune system then generates specific IgE antibodies that are like custom-made keys designed to fit that particular food allergen. These IgE antibodies attach themselves to specific immune cells called *mast cells*, which are found throughout the body's tissues, particularly in areas exposed to the environment such as the skin, gut, and respiratory tract. These IgE antibodies also attach to basophils that circulate in the bloodstream. This process of allergic sensitization *primes* the immune system, meaning it is on a high state of alert, for future exposure to the allergen.

The allergic reaction

The next time the person encounters the offending food, the allergenic proteins bind to the IgE antibodies that are attached to mast cells and basophils causing

IgE crosslinking. The crosslinking of IgE antibodies on the mast cell and basophil sends instructions to the mast cell and basophil causing activation and release of the cell's inflammatory chemicals, a process known as *degranulation.*

These inflammatory chemicals (which include tryptase, histamine, leukotrienes, and prostaglandins) work together to stimulate the dilation of blood vessels (a process known as *vasodilation*), causing smooth muscles to contract, and increasing the production of mucus, all of which leads to the classic symptoms of food allergy.

This sequence of events is known as the *allergic cascade.* The associated food allergy symptoms that follow can range from mild to severe and, in the case of anaphylaxis, can even be life-threatening.

Diagnosing Adverse Food Reactions

In order to diagnose your adverse food reactions, your physician should take a detailed medical history and conduct a physical examination. Your physician may also ask you about the specific details of your reaction to narrow the range of suspected food triggers that may cause your reaction. The following steps can help both you and your physician more accurately identify what is triggering your food allergy and when your symptoms are more likely to occur.

Keeping a food diary

TIP

A detailed food diary, in which you record everything you consume (even those midnight snacks) and describe your reactions, can help your physician diagnose your condition.

A well-kept food diary can assist you in telling your physician about the following items:

>> The timing of your reactions. For example, do they occur immediately after you've consumed a food or liquid, and if not, how long afterward?

>> The amount of food that seems to trigger a reaction.

>> The duration and severity of your symptoms.

>> Any activities, especially exercise, associated with your reactions.

Considering atopic causes

As part of the physical examination, your physician should also look for signs of atopic diseases, including

>> Dry, scaly skin, which can indicate atopic dermatitis

>> Dark circles under your eyes, which may indicate allergic rhinitis

>> Wheezing and coughing, which can signal asthma symptoms

Eliminating possible food culprits

In some cases, your physician may advise an *elimination diet* for you as a way of confirming what triggers your adverse reactions. This process involves eliminating suspected foods from your diet, one at a time, under your physician's supervision. If your symptoms significantly improve, your physician may then gradually reintroduce the likeliest food suspect to determine whether it's the source of your woes.

SEE YOUR DOCTOR

Only undergo an elimination diet under the direction of a physician. You don't want to deprive yourself of foods that may not cause your symptoms and are vital for your well-being. In fact, unsupervised elimination diets could result in nutritional deficiencies. Your physician may also advise an elimination diet in order to prepare you for an oral food challenge, which we describe in the next section.

Testing for food allergens

If your physician can't readily identify the cause of your reactions, they may also recommend confirming a suspected food allergen with the allergy tests that we describe in the following sections.

Skin testing

Skin testing involves using specific food extracts to evaluate your sensitivity to suspected allergens. Only a qualified specialist, such as an allergist, should perform skin testing. Skin testing for food allergens isn't always recommended.

WARNING

In some cases, your physician may not advise skin testing because a positive reaction may involve unacceptable risks of inducing anaphylactic shock, particularly if you're highly sensitized to certain foods, such as peanuts.

In general, prick-puncture tests are the only skin tests that your physician needs to administer when attempting to identify suspected food allergens. *Intracutaneous tests* (small injections of weakened allergen extract just under the surface of the skin on the patient's arm) are rarely advisable in these cases. (See Chapter 3 if you're on pins and needles about prick-puncture tests.)

Oral food challenges

Oral food challenges involve actually ingesting — under medical supervision — minute quantities of food that contain suspected allergens.

To ensure the most accurate diagnosis, your physician should administer an oral food challenge while you're symptom-free, usually as a result of a food elimination diet. Depending on the severity of your adverse food reactions and the type of food allergen that your physician suspects as the cause, your physician may choose to administer one of more of the following types of oral food challenges:

SEE YOUR DOCTOR

>> **Open challenge:** In this type of test, your physician informs you of what type of food you're ingesting so that both of you are aware that you're consuming the food allergen.

>> **Single-blind challenge:** With this test, you aren't told what you're fed. However, your physician or the clinician administering the test knows the ingredients.

>> **Double-blind, placebo-controlled oral food challenge (DBPCOFC):** This elaborate procedure is the gold standard for identifying food allergens. Neither you nor your physician (nor the clinician who administers the test) knows the contents of the test. In most cases, your physician schedules a DBPCOFC so you can fast for a prescribed amount of time beforehand. The initial dose of the suspected food in this type of challenge is usually half of the minimum quantity that your physician estimates as the trigger for your reaction.

As in all allergic challenges, you'll need to stop taking antihistamines (based on your physician's advice) prior to the challenge, because these drugs can interfere with the accuracy of this diagnostic procedure.

WARNING

Take this challenge only in a facility equipped to treat potentially severe reactions. If your history of adverse food reactions is life-threatening, your physician will most likely advise you that an oral food challenge is too risky.

ImmunoCAP

Your physician may advise using ImmunoCAP, which is a blood test that uses fluorescently labeled detection antibodies to measure levels of specific IgEs.

Although ImmunoCAP isn't as precise, practical, comprehensive, or cost-effective as allergy skin testing, your physician may recommend this procedure under specific circumstances. See Chapter 3 for more information on ImmunoCAP.

Basophil activation test (BAT)

The basophil activation test (BAT) is a laboratory assay that's currently being investigated for its potential to diagnose allergies. It works by measuring the response of basophils when exposed to a suspected allergen. During an allergic reaction, basophils release inflammatory mediators, such as histamine, during degranulation. The BAT detects signs of this chemical release using flow cytometry. At the present time, the use of the BAT is largely restricted to clinical research. However, it's showing promising results and may soon have utility as another diagnostic tool for the evaluation of food allergy.

Avoiding Adverse Food Reactions

After your physician determines the source of your adverse food reactions the most effective long-term approach to managing your condition and preventing further reactions is strict avoidance of the implicated food. That may seem like an obvious solution. However, you may need to become an expert at reading ingredient listings when you buy groceries. In some cases, food allergens and other types of precipitants may hide under arcane names in food labels. For updates and information on food allergens and related issues and to find out how to decipher ingredients listed on food labels, contact Food Allergy Research & Education (FARE) www.foodallergy.org.

You should make sure that your family, friends, and colleagues all understand what causes your adverse food reactions. You can then minimize the chances of erupting in hives at the Thanksgiving meal or during that crucial dinner with your boss and the company's new clients.

TIP

If you have life-threatening food hypersensitivity, you may need to avoid certain restaurants. In many cases, food servers don't have enough information about the ingredients in the establishment's menu to guarantee you an allergen-free meal, although some restaurants actually do offer dishes without common food allergens. However, we strongly advise double-checking all the ingredients in the menu item with the chef or restaurant manager. In particular, you need to inquire whether the restaurant prepares allergen-free meals using surfaces, cookware, and utensils that are separated from the other items in the kitchen.

If effective management of your adverse food reactions involves excluding common food groups from your diet for long periods, consider professional dietary advice and ask your physician to refer you to a dietitian, in order to prevent nutritional deficiency or malnutrition.

Treating Food Allergy

If you (or your loved one) suffer from food allergies, and you're reading this book, you probably know that no real cure for food allergy currently exists. The cornerstone of managing the food allergy involves strict avoidance of the offending food(s) and the use of rescue medication (epinephrine) in the event of accidental exposure.

Thanks to several new treatments being developed to treat food allergies, the future looks bright for food allergy sufferers and their families. Although some of the new treatment options may take a few years to become widely available, they offer hope for more choices and personalized care. That means that food allergy sufferers will be able to proactively partner with their physician in a process known as shared decision making, to find a treatment plan that best fits their individual needs.

The following sections describe the current treatments that are available for food allergies and share some exciting news on what's on the horizon in the quest for new food allergy treatments.

Examining allergen immunotherapy (AIT)

This treatment approach for food allergies has become popular in recent years. It involves gradually exposing the allergic person to the allergen over time using one of the following four approaches.

Oral immunotherapy (OIT)

OIT is a treatment for food allergies that involves the person with a specific food allergy gradually eating small amounts of the allergenic protein daily. Doing so helps to retrain the immune system to tolerate the food allergen and reduces the risk of a severe reaction due to accidental ingestion.

In 2020, the FDA approved Palforzia, the first treatment for peanut allergy only, in children 4 to 17 years of age and very recently it has been approved down to 1 year of age. Palforzia consists of purified peanut protein that is ingested, starting with a minute amount of the protein powder, gradually building up to a maintenance dose that is to be eaten daily.

Research has shown that over time, consuming Palforzia helps to desensitize the person with a peanut allergy and offers *bite protection* in the event that they accidentally ingest peanut protein. However, Palforzia doesn't offer complete protection from accidental exposure to peanuts, and an allergic reaction may still occur. Therefore, continuing to avoid peanuts and carrying rescue medication (for instance, epinephrine) is essential.

Sublingual immunotherapy (SLIT)

This form of immunotherapy involves dissolving the food allergen in a small amount of liquid and then having the person with the allergy hold it under their tongue for several minutes before spitting out the mixture. The undigested allergen interacts with the immune cells in the lining of the mouth, gradually reducing the person's sensitivity to the food allergen and improving tolerance over time. Although this treatment has shown promising results in clinical trials, the FDA hasn't approved it, and it's still only available in clinical research.

Oral mucosal immunotherapy (OMIT)

Oral mucosal immunotherapy (OMIT) is a new delivery platform being evaluated for the treatment of food allergies. The process involves embedding the allergen (for example, peanut) into a fully functional toothpaste that can be conveniently administered as a daily treatment while patients brush their teeth. The process of tooth brushing allows the food allergen to interact with the immune cells in the mouth, resulting in the gradual buildup of tolerance over time. OMIT has shown promising results in a recent clinical trial, and more research is being conducted to achieve FDA approval.

Epicutaneous immunotherapy (EPIT)

Epicutaneous immunotherapy (EPIT) involves delivering the food allergen through the skin of the person with the allergy, using a Viaskin EPIT patch. It's designed to induce an immune response in the patient over time by introducing minimal amounts of allergen to the skin. The patch is placed onto the skin daily to make the patient less sensitive to their food allergen. It's currently being investigated for the treatment of peanut, egg, and milk allergy. The Viaskin peanut patch specifically, is under FDA review, but hasn't been approved as of this writing.

Reaching a new treatment horizon: Biologics

Biologic medications are drugs that target specific part of your immune systems to treat disease. They're human made proteins that are designed to affect the parts of the immune system that trigger inflammation and treat diseases such as asthma, atopic dermatitis, eosinophilic inflammation and nasal polyps. These medicines are usually given as an injection or as an infusion into a vein.

These medications represent a new approach for the development of treatments that inhibit specific mechanisms of food allergy. Presently, biologics, and in particular anti-lgE, are being investigated for the possible treatment of food allergies.

The FDA has recently approved omalizumab (Xolair) for the treatment of multiple food allergies — including peanut, milk, egg, wheat, cashew, and shellfish — in persons aged 1 to 55. Xolair is injected subcutaneously (under the skin) every 2 to 4 weeks. The dose of Xolair is dependent upon the weight and starting IgE level of the allergic person.

Xolair works by binding IgE antibodies, preventing them from attaching to mast cells and basophils, thus inhibiting the allergic reaction. This reduces the body's sensitivity to the allergens, lessening the risk and severity of allergic reactions upon accidental exposure.

The approval of Xolair as a new treatment for food allergy is a welcome development particularly for individuals with multiple, severe food allergies and/or other comorbid allergic conditions such as asthma or urticaria (hives). Under certain conditions Xolair has the potential to be used as an adjunct to immunotherapy in patients with single and multiple food allergies, enabling them to reach their maintenance dose more rapidly and safely, by reducing the risks associated with increasing dosages.

Note: Xolair isn't a disease-modifying agent. That means that if individuals with allergies stop receiving their frequent injections, their food allergy is likely to return within a short period of time. Therefore, lifelong treatment may be required.

Thanks to ongoing research in the United States and around the world, we're hopeful that additional treatments for food allergy will be available in the near future.

PREVENTING FOOD ALLERGIES?
YES OR NO?

Did you know that new evidence is emerging that food allergies might be preventable?

Until very recently the standard practice of avoiding major food allergens in the first year of life, was considered the gold standard for preventing food allergies. However recent research is largely turning this on its head and is now advocating exactly the opposite, recommending that food allergens should actually be introduced to babies' diets during the early months of life.

This paradigm shift in scientific thinking, resulted from landmark studies like the LEAP (Learning Early About Peanut Allergy) and EAT (Enquiring About Tolerance) trials, which provide strong evidence that introducing certain food allergens, like peanut and egg, between 4 to 11 months of age, significantly reduces the risk of developing food allergies in later life. The hypothesis suggests that introducing these allergenic food proteins early in a baby's life may help to educate the immature immune system to tolerate the potential allergen, thereby preventing future food allergies.

Although these findings are very promising, we'd caution that this approach doesn't have proven success for all allergens, (such as milk, for example) and more research is needed. However, the evidence supporting the early introduction of peanut and egg, in particular, is so compelling, that both the American Academy of Pediatrics and the National Institute of Allergy and Infectious Diseases (NIAID) have updated their recommendations regarding the early introduction of these foods for infants. If you're a parent, make sure to discuss these new strategies with your pediatrician to determine the best approach for your child.

Chapter **16**

Diagnosing and Treating Drug Reactions

The term *wonder drug* is an apt description of the benefits that many modern-day medications provide. These products — such as antibiotics, insulin, anti-inflammatories, biologics, and other drugs — enable physicians to treat or cure conditions that once seemed beyond remedy. When prescribed and used properly, most of these medications — such as the ones we discuss for treating nasal allergies (see Part 2) and asthma (see Part 3) — cause few if any serious side effects.

However, adverse drug reactions are a concern for some people. Although these reactions occur much less frequently than the known potential side effects that you may hear about at the end of a medication's television commercial, adverse drug reactions account for as many as 100,000 deaths in the United States each year, according to recent estimates.

Any unexpected adverse consequence of taking medication, other than for the purpose that it's intended, is considered to be an adverse drug reaction. This definition doesn't include intentional or accidental poisoning, drug abuse, overdose, or treatment failures.

Patients most at risk for adverse drug reactions include those who have

>> Serious illnesses that require high doses and/or many types of medications.

>> Impaired liver and kidney functions, especially patients who consume large quantities of alcohol.

>> Compromised immune systems, especially individuals with HIV/AIDS. In these cases, the drugs most likely to cause adverse reactions are sulfadiazine (Silvadene), acyclovir (Zovirax), and zidovudine (Retrovir).

Understanding Adverse Drug Reactions

Adverse drug reactions can be classified as those that are predictable and those that are unpredictable. (We discuss unpredictable reactions in the section "Under-standing Drug Intolerance and Idiosyncrasy" later in this chapter.)

Predictable adverse drug reactions include the following:

>> **Known side effects:** The product information package inserts that accompany all types of medications list these types of reactions. For example, a typical side effect of aspirin in some people is stomach irritation, and a frequent side effect of many first-generation over-the-counter (OTC) antihistamines (such as Benadryl) is drowsiness.

>> **Drug interactions:** As we explain in Chapters 3 and 6, always make sure that any physician who treats you knows about any and all products you take for other medical conditions. This list includes any OTC drugs you may take, even for minor aches and pains, as well as any vitamins and nutritional supplements. Some of these drugs don't work well together, as we explain in these two examples:

- If you have asthma and are also taking oral beta-blockers such as Inderal, Lopressor, and Corgard (for migraine headaches, high blood pressure, angina, or hyperthyroidism) or beta-blocker eyedrops such as Timoptic (for glaucoma), these medications might block the effect of your inhaled short-acting adrenergic bronchodilator, thus depriving you of quick relief when you need it for respiratory symptoms. Occasionally, taking beta-blockers can trigger asthma episodes in susceptible individuals who haven't previously experienced any respiratory symptoms.

- Drug combinations may also result in other serious consequences. For example, if you take fluconazole (Diflucan) (which some physicians use to treat some cases of fungal infections) and then also take prescribed erythromycin (an antibiotic) for a bacterial infection, the combined effects of these two drugs may impair your liver's ability to metabolize and clear erythromycin from your system. Combining these medications can increase the risk of an irregular heart rhythm (an *arrhythmia*) that could be potentially life-threatening.

>> **Accidental or intentional overdose:** Remember, too much of anything can be bad for you. Use only products and preparations — whether prescription or OTC — that are clearly labeled to treat the symptoms you're experiencing. Also, always carefully read the product information package insert and take the medication only as the label or your doctor instructs.

Adverse drug reactions can also be defined according to the mechanisms that cause them, although doctors don't yet fully understand what makes some of us react to certain drugs in certain ways. The following three sections explain these mechanisms.

Drug hypersensitivities

REMEMBER

Also known as drug allergies, *drug hypersensitivities* involve specific immunologic responses (see Chapter 2) to certain drugs in people who have developed allergic sensitivities to allergenic substances in these drugs. The most frequent type of adverse allergic reactions to medications occurs with penicillin and its related compounds. Other drugs that can cause allergic reactions include cephalosporins, sulfonamides, insulin, and anti-sera (horse serum for anti-venom treatment of snake bites).

Aspirin, OTC nonsteroidal anti-inflammatory drugs (NSAIDs) such as ibuprofen (Advil, Motrin), ketoprofen (Actron, Orudis), naproxen (Aleve), and sometimes newer prescription NSAIDs, known as COX-2 inhibitors — including celecoxib (Celebrex) and meloxicam (Mobic) — and other drugs can also trigger adverse reactions. However, these reactions aren't truly considered allergic because in most cases, immunologic mechanisms aren't involved.

Non-immunologic drug reactions

Most adverse drug reactions are *non-immunologic* — not involving any of the four types of immunologic processes that we explain in Chapter 2. Aspirin and NSAIDs are the main culprits in these types of reactions, which include the following categories:

>> **Drug idiosyncrasy:** An unexpected and unpredictable effect that doesn't relate to the intended action of the drug (for example, severe anemia

occurring in certain groups of people, after taking medications such as anti-malarials, sulfonamides, and pain relievers).

>> **Drug intolerance:** An undesirable effect that occurs at lower-than-normal doses of a drug, for which no scientific explanation has yet been discovered. For example, *tinnitus* (ringing in the ears) can occur in some individuals after taking just a single aspirin tablet.

Pseudoallergic drug reactions

Pseudoallergic drug reactions often mimic drug hypersensitivity reactions and can result in anaphylaxis. These reactions aren't truly the result of an immuno-logic mechanism involving IgE antibodies (agents that cause the release of inflammatory chemicals such as histamine from the mast cells that line tissues in many parts of the body, thus inducing allergy symptoms), but a response similar to drug hypersensitivity occurs, nonetheless. They usually produce these allergic-like responses by directly binding to cells like mast cells without the need to involve IgE. This direct binding causes the mast cell, for example, to release the same chemicals as are released in the immunologic reaction utilizing IgE as the cell binding intermediary, the immunologic mechanism.

WARNING

If you're susceptible to a pseudoallergic reaction from a particular drug, you may have an immediate and severe reaction the very first time you use the substance instead of after more than one exposure to allergenic substances in the drug, as is the case with true hypersensitivities or allergies.

REMEMBER

Aspirin and NSAIDs are also often implicated in pseudoallergic cases. Other medications that can produce pseudoallergic reactions include the following:

>> Radio-contrast media (RCM), containing organic iodine, used in some diagnos-tic tests, such as intravenous pyelogram (IVP) to check for kidney and urinary tract problems

>> Colloid volume substitutes (used for severe cases of shock) such as dextran, gelatin, hydroxyethel starch, and human serum albumin

>> Opiates such as codeine, meperidine, and morphine prescribed for pain management

Identifying Forms of Drug Hypersensitivities

Contrary to popular belief, only a small number of adverse drug reactions occur as a result of drug hypersensitivities (also known as drug allergies).

Drug hypersensitivities can develop if you've been sensitized to one of the otherwise harmless components of a drug. As a result, your immune system produces agents (known as IgE antibodies) as a response to these allergens. The more exposure you receive to a drug that may trigger an allergic response, the greater chance you have for developing a hypersensitivity to that substance (see Chapter 2 for an extensive explanation of this process).

Factors that determine your risk of developing a drug hypersensitivity can include

>> The dosage level of your medication

>> How the drug is administered — orally, topically, via injection, or intravenously (IV)

>> How long you take the drug

>> How many courses of the drug you've taken before

>> Other concurrent illnesses you many have, such as asthma, cystic fibrosis, mononucleosis, human immunodeficiency virus (HIV/AIDS, in addition to the ailment for which your doctor prescribes the drug

>> Your age, gender, and family history

The following sections provide greater detail about drug hypersensitivities.

SKIN SENSITIZING AND DRUG ALLERGIES

While medicating your skin, you may also sensitize your body to substances that a topical product contains. This problem frequently occurs with ethylenediamine (EDA), a chemical that has been widely used as a stabilizer in topical anti-infective medications, such as Mycolog-II Cream and similar generic products.

We strongly advise against using topical forms — whether in prescription or OTC strengths — of antibiotics (such as neomycin), local anesthetics (such as benzocaine), and antihistamines (such as Benadryl and Caladry) without first asking your physician. You could develop a sensitivity to the substances in these topical preparations, which can subsequently result in a potentially serious systemic reaction if you take the drug in an oral or injected form.

Recognizing signs of drug hypersensitivities

Certain drugs tend to produce reactions in specific tissues and organs. Although drug hypersensitivity reactions most frequently target the skin, the reaction can affect any organ system in your body, including mucous membranes, lymph nodes, kidneys, liver, lungs, and joints.

Common signs of allergic reactions that affect various organs and functions include the following symptoms:

>> **Skin rashes:** Allergic drug rashes, which often take the form of red, itchy bumps, may appear all over your body. If a topical drug causes the reaction, the rash usually appears at the site where you applied the product. However, you may also have a reaction on your hands or any other part of your body that came into contact with the product. (See Chapter 11 for more on topical drugs and contact dermatitis.)

>> **Urticaria (hives) and angioedema (deep swelling):** These red, itchy welts and swollen lesions can appear anywhere on your body as a systemic allergic reaction to certain drugs. The most frequent allergic triggers of urticaria and angioedema for sensitized people include penicillin, sulfonamides, cephalosporins, insulin, and anti-sera (such as horse serum). Pseudoallergic reactions, frequently caused by aspirin, NSAIDs, and narcotic pain relievers, also commonly trigger hives and angioedema.

>> **Other skin reactions:** In rare cases, more serious skin conditions can result from adverse allergic drug reactions. These more serious conditions can include

- **Exfoliative dermatitis:** This potentially life-threatening reaction may cause the top skin layer of your skin to shed over much of your body, with the remaining layer becoming red and scaly.

- **Erythema multiforme:** This widespread reaction can produce itchy rashes on many parts of your body, most characteristically on the backs of your hands and feet. Very often, the hallmark pattern of this eruption resembles a bull's-eye, or in medicalese, a *target* or *iris lesion*. In many cases, you may also have a headache and fever.

- **Stevens-Johnson syndrome:** This extremely rare but serious condition can produce substantial tissue damage, often involving mucous membranes, such as your mouth, throat, and eyes. The reaction can also target internal organs such as your liver, kidney, and lungs. This syndrome can also result from a nonallergic, viral-precipitating factor, especially a herpes simplex infection.

- >> **Internal organs and functions:** Adverse drug reactions can also affect the lungs, liver, kidneys, gastrointestinal tract, and mucous membranes. Reactions involving your lungs may trigger asthma symptoms, such as wheezing, or can lead to pneumonia.

- >> **Fever:** In some patients, an allergic drug reaction may also cause a *drug fever*, occasionally accompanied by shaking, chills, and a skin rash.

- >> **Blood:** In some cases, adverse drug reactions can destroy and impair your body's ability to produce red blood cells, leading to low blood pressure and/or anemia.

- >> **Anaphylaxis:** In less frequent, but more serious cases, an immunologic adverse drug reaction can result in *anaphylaxis*, a severe, potentially life-threatening response that affects many organs simultaneously. According to recent estimates, anaphylaxis from penicillin hypersensitivity is the leading cause of drug-related anaphylactic deaths in the United States, usually due to injections of penicillin. Fortunately, the use of penicillin shots has significantly decreased in recent years.

TECHNICAL STUFF

WHAT'S ACETYL GOT TO DO WITH HIVES?

Aspirin (acetylsalicylic acid) is one of the most common triggers of hives. Although hives and angioedema are inflammatory conditions, you generally shouldn't take acetylated forms of aspirin or other related anti-inflammatory medications to relieve these conditions without first consulting your physician. This advice also applies to OTC nonsteroidal anti-inflammatory drugs (NSAIDs), most of which contain ibuprofen (Advil, Motrin), ketoprofen (Actron, Orudis), or naproxen (Aleve) as active ingredients, and sometimes, newer prescription NSAIDs, known as COX-2 inhibitors — including celecoxib (Celebrex) and meloxicam (Mobic). Likewise, avoid combination pain relievers that include any of these active ingredients.

In many cases, you can use acetaminophen (Tylenol) or salicylsalicylic acid (Disalcid, Salflex), a non-acetylated form of aspirin known as *salsalate*, as substitutes for acetylated aspirin and NSAIDs. COX-2 inhibitors may often be used as a substitute when NSAIDs are needed.

Explaining mechanisms of drug hypersensitivity

Your immune system can respond to different types of allergens in a variety of ways. Although drug hypersensitivities can involve all four types of immune system mechanisms (see Chapter 2), in most allergic reactions, one mechanism usually predominates.

The following section explains various mechanisms of drug hypersensitivities:

» **IgE-medicated reactions (Type I):** This category of hypersensitivity results in immediate reactions such as anaphylaxis and includes symptoms of hives, swelling of the throat, wheezing, and cardiorespiratory collapse. The most common culprits for this extreme drug reaction are penicillin and its relatives. If you've had a prior allergic reaction to penicillin, you're six times more likely than the general population to experience another severe allergic reaction if you take this antibiotic again.

» **Cytotoxic reactions (Type II):** These reactions are serious and potentially life-threatening. They involve cell destruction, possibly resulting in the breakdown of your red blood cells, leading to anemia and decreased numbers of platelets in your blood (needed to make your blood clot). Drugs known to cause these reactions include penicillin, sulfonamides (Bactrim, Septra), and quinidine (Apo-Quinidine, Quinalan).

» **Immune complex reactions (Type III):** Manifestations of this reaction include fever, rash, hives, and symptoms that affect the lymph nodes and joints. This reaction, which physicians refer to as *serum sickness*, typically appears one to three weeks after taking the final doses of drugs such as penicillin, sulfonamides, thiouracil, and phenytoin.

» **Cell-mediated reactions (Type IV):** Contact dermatitis is the primary sign of this localized, nonsystemic reaction (see Chapter 12). In cell-mediated reactions, symptoms appear on your skin after using topical drug preparations to which you're sensitized. The most frequent medication causes of this reaction are topical antibiotic preparations such as neomycin (Neosporin), topical anesthetics such as benzocaine and other -caines (Lanacane, Solarcaine), and antihistamines such as diphenhydramine (Benadryl).

Understanding Drug Intolerance and Idiosyncrasy

Unlike drug hypersensitivities, the production and interaction of IgE antibodies by your immune system aren't factors in drug *idiosyncrasy* (medicalese for "we don't know") and drug intolerance reactions. For this reason, these types of reactions are far less predictable than those that result from drug hypersensitivities. Although the mechanisms involved in these kinds of reactions are less well documented, most adverse drug reactions fall into this category.

REMEMBER

The drugs most often associated with drug idiosyncrasy and drug intolerance include

» **Quinidine:** Even a small dose of this medication, prescribed for arrhythmia (irregular heartbeat), can lead to tinnitus in some heart patients.

» **Aspirin and NSAIDs, sometimes including newer prescription NSAIDs, known as COX-2 inhibitors:** If you're an asthma patient with nasal polyps and an aspirin sensitivity, using these pain relievers or related anti-inflammatories can lead to the potentially serious and even life-threatening symptoms of severe *bronchoconstriction* (constricted airways). This syndrome is known as *aspirin-exacerbated respiratory disease (AERD)* — asthma, nasal polyps, aspirin sensitivity, and a history of sinusitis — which we explain more extensively in Chapter 9.

» **Angiotensin-converting enzyme (ACE) inhibitors:** These inhibitors can produce coughing and angioedema. The coughing usually disappears within several weeks of discontinuing ACE medications. However, angioedema resulting from use of these medications can cause life-threatening complications, sometimes requiring hospitalization.

Other symptoms of non-immunologic aspirin and NSAID drug reactions can include generalized urticaria (total body hives), *rhinoconjunctivitis* (inflammation of the nasal passages and eyes), and airway *edema* (swelling of the airways).

Diagnosing Adverse Drug Reactions

Diagnosing adverse drug reactions — such as suspicious rash, fever, swollen and tender lymph nodes, or lung, kidney, or gastrointestinal disturbances — soon after starting a new drug can present a challenge. In fact, the testing options for determining whether an allergic mechanism causes your reactions are limited.

In most cases, your medical history is the most important factor in making an accurate diagnosis. The next section outline the key steps you and your physician can take to help accurately diagnose your adverse drug reaction.

Taking your drug reaction history

SEE YOUR DOCTOR

To evaluate the likelihood of an adverse drug reaction as the cause of the types of symptoms, your doctor needs to take a thorough medical history. Be prepared to provide your doctor with detailed information about your medication use, because the physician probably needs to ask questions such as the following:

» What drugs are you currently using and what drugs have you taken in the past?

» How long did you take a particular drug before symptoms started?

» Have you had similar episodes in the past?

» Has anyone in your family experienced adverse drug reactions?

Keeping track of your drugs

TIP

Determining the source of your adverse drug reactions can prove particularly tricky when you take more than one medication. Keeping a symptom diary can enable you to help your doctor narrow down the likeliest causes of your adverse reactions. (In Chapter 3, we discuss this topic in greater detail.)

In addition to a symptom diary, we also recommend establishing a drug record that lists all the medications — prescription and/or OTC — you have taken over your lifetime. Think of this diary as similar to recording your workout training schedule.

TIP

Your drug record should include information such as the following:

» The brand and generic names of all the drugs, both prescription and over the counter (OTC), you've used and are currently taking

» A list of all supplements, including any vitamins, minerals, pre and probiotics and alternative herbal remedies that you are currently taking

» The conditions you're treating or have treated with particular drugs

» The effectiveness and/or results of taking these drugs

>> For prescription products, the names of the physicians who prescribed those drugs and the dates when you received the prescription

>> Any side effects and/or adverse reactions you may have experienced while taking the drugs

Undergoing diagnostic testing for drug hypersensitivities

Allergy skin testing can prove helpful for diagnosing allergies to a few drugs, such as penicillin and related antibiotics, insulin, local anesthetics, and vaccines. Skin testing for these drugs should only be done if your doctor considers these products essential for treating a medical condition that severely affects you and if your medical history indicates a likelihood of anaphylactic reactions to these medications.

For the majority of patients who have experienced less severe, non-anaphylactic reactions, drug challenges are considered to be the standard for determining tolerance to a medication. Drug challenges may be given in an incremental fashion but can also be administered as a single dose depending on the patient's medical history.

WARNING

Skin testing isn't advisable if penicillin and related antibiotics are implicated in a previous, severe, non-immunologic systemic reaction, such as exfoliative dermatitis, erythema multiforme, or Stevens-Johnson syndrome (see "Recognizing signs of drug hypersensitivities" earlier in this chapter). For an in-depth discussion of allergy skin testing, see Chapter 6.

Using patch testing for drug reactions

For cases involving cell-mediated reactions, such as localized, non-systemic reactions to topical preparations (characteristic of contact dermatitis), patch testing is the gold standard for diagnosing drug hypersensitivities.

Patch testing involves applying patches that contain small amounts of suspected allergens directly to your skin. A positive reaction usually appears as a small area of allergic contact dermatitis within one to four days (see Chapter 12 for more information on contact dermatitis).

WARNING

If you have a severe or widespread outbreak of contact dermatitis, we don't advise using a patch test. Your doctor should also instruct you to immediately remove any patch that causes severe irritation.

Exploring general clinical testing for drug reactions

For cases involving potential late-phase drug hypersensitivity reactions that appear days or weeks after you take a particular medication, your doctor may advise other types of clinical testing. These tests can include the following:

>> In the event that lung and/or heart complications develop days or weeks after starting a drug, your doctor may advise a chest X-ray and/or electrocardiogram (EKG).

>> If your doctor suspects that an adverse drug reaction may affect your liver or kidneys, they may advise tests for those organ functions.

>> If your doctor suspects a cytotoxic reaction, they may advise complete blood and platelet counts.

>> If a suspected adverse drug reaction involves symptoms such as drug fever (see "Recognizing signs of drug hypersensitivities" earlier in this chapter), *eosinophilic pneumonia* (a form of pneumonia that features nonproductive coughing as the main symptom and is characterized by elevated eosinophils; see Chapter 2), or an immune system disorder, your doctor may advise further tests to confirm the diagnosis.

Reducing Adverse Drug Reaction Risks

Your best bet for managing adverse drug reactions, as with other kinds of allergies, consists of avoiding the problematic substances. Using medication — particularly topical drugs — only when you really need them, instead of resorting to products and preparations for every ache and pain, can reduce your risks of developing drug sensitivities.

REMEMBER

In addition, the overuse of antibiotics, especially for inappropriate treatment of viral infections such as the common cold and flu (for which antibiotics are ineffective), contributes to an increased incidence of drug sensitivity throughout the world.

Treating your reactions

For mild reactions, simply stopping the drug in question is the best remedy. When you experience more severe symptoms, your doctor may institute drug therapy to counteract your adverse reaction.

Drug therapy usually involves using one or more antihistamines, such as hydroxyzine (Atarax) and/or diphenhydramine (Benadryl), as well as a short course of oral corticosteroids (especially for symptoms such as persistent joint inflammation and discomfort) if needed. For pain, physicians often recommend acetaminophen (Tylenol) as the first choice, a nonacetylated form of aspirin, known as *salsalate*, such as salicylsalicylic acid (Disalcid, Salflex) or a COX-2 inhibitor such as celecoxib (Celebrex) or meloxicam (Mobic).

Managing severe adverse drug reactions

If an adverse reaction causes severe skin problems, such as rashes, hives, or angioedema, or if you experience drug-induced anemia or platelet problems, your doctor may advise a short course of oral corticosteroids.

A life-threatening reaction such as anaphylaxis usually requires immediate administration of epinephrine (adrenaline), oxygen, antihistamines, and corticosteroids.

SEE YOUR
DOCTOR

If you experience a non-immunologic adverse reaction to a drug that's essential for treating another medical condition from which you suffer, your doctor may treat you preventively with a short course of oral corticosteroids and antihistamines. This preventative treatment can often enable you to use the potentially problematic drug in the short term with a much-reduced risk of an adverse reaction.

WARNING

If your doctor determines that you may experience a serious adverse drug reaction to particular drugs, wear a MedicAlert tag or bracelet. If you're unable to communicate during a medical emergency, the information on the tag can prevent you from receiving an accidental dose of a drug that can trigger an adverse reaction.

Recently, the U.S. Food and Drug Administration approved the first non-injectable emergency treatment for anaphylaxis, in the form of a single dose epinephrine nasal spray called neffy. For more information on anaphylaxis and neffy, see Chapter 14.

Preventing penicillin problems

WARNING

Simply staying away from a specific drug may not sufficiently eliminate your adverse drug reaction. If you're allergic to penicillin, you also need to avoid other antibiotic relatives of this drug, including frequently prescribed antibiotics such as ampicillin and amoxicillin. In addition, some patients with penicillin sensitivities may cross-react with certain cephalosporin antibiotics.

MISLABELED PENICILLIN ALLERGIES

The majority of penicillin reactions are self-reported and actually inconsistent with a true allergy. Most reported penicillin allergy symptoms are nonimmediate dermatologic symptoms that occurred at a young age during the first or early part of the second week of oral treatment, usually with amoxicillin.

Unfortunately, patients with this mislabel of "penicillin allergy" are likely to be treated with less effective and more expensive antibiotics leading to increased costs and longer hospital stays. Penicillin allergy assessment to de-label inaccurate "penicillin allergy" should be done whenever possible.

TIP

If you experience an allergic reaction, such as a rash to an antibiotic, we suggest that you stop taking the medication (with your doctor's consent) and wait until your reaction resolves before starting another antibiotic as an immediate substitute. Many experts believe you're in a hypersensitive state during the period of time that an allergic reaction takes place, and you risk developing a sensitivity to another antibiotic if you begin taking it while your allergic symptoms are still present.

WARNING

If you develop a mild rash while taking an antibiotic such as amoxicillin/potassium clavulanate (Augmentin) for your sinusitis, your doctor may advise you to wait a few days or more (depending on the severity of your response) until the reaction resolves before you switch to an alternative, unrelated antibiotic, such as clarithromycin (Biaxin). Doing so may reduce the risk of sensitizing your immune system to other families of antibiotics.

Desensitizing your drug hypersensitivities

If you have a hypersensitivity to a medication that your doctor considers essential to your treatment, they may suggest skin testing, followed by rapid desensitization. The desensitization process requires rapidly administering incremental doses (starting with very small amounts) of the allergenic drug. The steady increase in dose desensitizes your immune system so that it doesn't trigger an allergic response when you get a therapeutic dose of the drug in question.

Desensitization should only be performed under the supervision of an experienced physician and in a medical facility equipped to handle emergency situations.

Chapter **17**

Preventing Insect Sting Reactions

nsect stings are a part of life. These creepy, crawly, and flying creatures have been around at least 400 million years (much longer than the human species), and they show no signs of going away. Although some insects spread diseases or harm crops, many of these creatures are essential and beneficial participants in the complex workings of the planet's ecosystems — for example, insects pollinate many crops, especially fruit.

However, if you're allergic to the venom from stinging insects, it can be a serious concern. This chapter is here to help. Here we identify common responses to insect stings, explore the main culprits that cause insect stings, discuss how insect hypersensitivities are diagnosed, and examine the ways to prevent, manage, and treat them when they do happen.

Getting the 4-1-1 on Insect Stings

Insect sting hypersensitivities are equal-opportunity allergies. Even if you have other allergic conditions — such as allergic rhinitis (hay fever), asthma, atopic dermatitis (eczema), or food allergies — or have a family history of *atopy* (a genetic susceptibility to developing allergic disease), you aren't at any greater risk than anyone else for having an allergic reaction to *Hymenoptera* insects.

WARNING

However, if you have a chronic heart or lung condition (such as coronary artery disease or asthma) and also have a stinging insect hypersensitivity, you may be at greater risk for developing more serious reactions if one of those creatures stings you.

Here we examine the types of reactions you may get from insect stings and the types of insect stings that can cause these reactions.

Reacting to insect stings

Insect stings usually produce only local nonallergic reactions, such as redness, itching, swelling, and pain, due to the potent chemicals contained in their venom. However, according to recent estimates, 3 percent of adults and 1 percent of children in the United States may be at risk for serious allergic reactions to certain insect stings, potentially resulting in the following types of systemic symptoms:

>> Hives (on your skin — not the ones where bees live), itching, and skin swellings on parts of your body other than the sting site — for example, more than just a large local reaction

>> *Bronchospasm* (airway constriction), tightness of the chest, and difficulty breathing

>> Hoarseness and swelling of the tongue, throat, and upper airway (laryngeal edema)

>> Dizziness

>> Hypotensive shock (sudden drop in blood pressure)

>> *Anaphylaxis* (a potentially life-threatening reaction affecting many organs simultaneously) occurs when all these symptoms occur together

Sting reactions are classified according to the type and severity of symptoms they produce. Here's what you need to know:

>> **Small, local reactions:** Most insect stings cause localized reactions that pose few serious medical consequences and don't require special treatment. However, you may experience redness, itching, swelling, and pain for several days at the sting site. Irritating enzymes and chemicals in insect venom, rather than an allergic mechanism, create these reactions.

>> **Large, local reactions:** These reactions involve extreme swelling that extends from the sting site, sometimes affecting an entire arm of leg. However, the swelling usually disappears in two to three days. As with small, local reactions, these large, local reactions result from the enzymes and chemicals in the insect's venom. You're at no greater risk than the general population of developing a serious, systemic reaction to an insect sting if you've ever experienced a large local reaction.

>> **Systemic reactions:** *Cutaneous* (skin-related) eruptions, such as *urticaria* (hives) and *angioedema* (deep swellings), over a large area of the body often are a feature of these more serious reactions. A systemic reaction results from an allergic mechanism. Unlike small or large local reactions, symptoms of a systemic reaction appear on areas of your body other than the sting site. After you've had one systemic reaction to a sting, you're likely to have the same or worse reaction if the same type of insect stings you again. However, treating the discomfort associated with these skin reactions is usually the only treatment necessary, because these symptoms are rarely life-threatening.

WARNING

>> **Life-threatening reactions:** Anaphylactic symptoms, such as swelling of the tongue and/or throat (laryngeal edema), breathing difficulty, and dizziness or fainting (due to a fall in blood pressure) are signs of this type of systemic reaction to insect venom. Approximately 70 people die each year in the United States from anaphylaxis resulting from severe allergic reactions to insect stings. If you experience a life-threatening reaction, you need immediate emergency treatment (refer to the section "Treating urgent insect sting cases," later in this chapter). In addition, because these potentially life-threatening reactions result from allergic triggers in the insect venom, your physician may recommend skin or blood testing and a course of venom immunotherapy (VIT) to prevent future reactions. (Read the section "Long-term treatment: Venom immunotherapy" later in this chapter for more information on VIT.)

Identifying what's bugging you

The stinging insects that can cause hypersensitivity reactions all belong to the *Hymenoptera* order — the third largest insect order — which encompasses more than 100,000 species. This insect order gets its name from Hymeno, the Greek god of marriage (whose name derives from the Greek word, "hymen," which means *membranous*), because the flying species of this order have two pairs of membranous front and back wings ("optera" in Greek), held together by tiny hooks so that they function as one unit (the way married couples are supposed to work).

The *Hymenoptera* insects responsible for producing allergic reactions belong to these three separate families:

>> **Apidae:** Honeybees are members of this family. Flowers and bright colors usually attract these busy bees. The bees in this family generally aren't aggressive, except for the Africanized honeybees (so-called killer bees).

>> **Vespidae:** This family includes yellow jackets, hornets, and wasps. These insects generally feed on human food, which is why you may see them hovering or crawling over garbage cans, leftover food on the picnic table, or at any outdoor event that includes food and sugary beverages.

>> **Formicidae:** These ant families include the two types of fire ants — red and black — that plague the southeastern U.S. and Puerto Rico and that are spreading throughout the rest of the southern states. These ants get their name from the painful, burning pustules that result from their (often) multiple stings. You certainly don't want these ants in your pants, or anywhere else in your vicinity, for that matter.

The good news is that although many insects bite or sting, only a very small percentage of stinging insects produce venom that can actually trigger allergic reactions. In fact, in terms of insect venom hypersensitivity, in the vast majority of cases, you only need to watch out for five groups of the estimated three million insect species, as shown in Figure 17-1:

>> Honeybees (bumblebees, which are solitary bees, are rare causes of insect sting reactions)

>> Yellow jackets

>> Wasps (specifically the social wasps, more commonly known as *paper wasps*)

>> Hornets (white faced and yellow hornets)

>> Fire ants (both the red and black species)

REMEMBER

Mosquitoes and other biting insects can cause painful and/or irritating bites and may also spread diseases, but they rarely cause severe allergic reactions. However, bites from genus *triatoma* (kissing bug or cone-nose bug, found primarily in rural areas of the southwestern United States) which are usually painless and almost always occur at night, have been associated with severe allergic reactions, including rare cases of anaphylaxis, due to the allergen contained in the insect's saliva.

On the other hand, you'll be happy to know that cross-reactivity is far more limited between the stinging insect families. For example, multiple sensitivity to both honeybees (Apids) and yellow jackets (Vespids) is much less common than multiple sensitivity to hornets and yellow jackets (both members of the Vespid family).

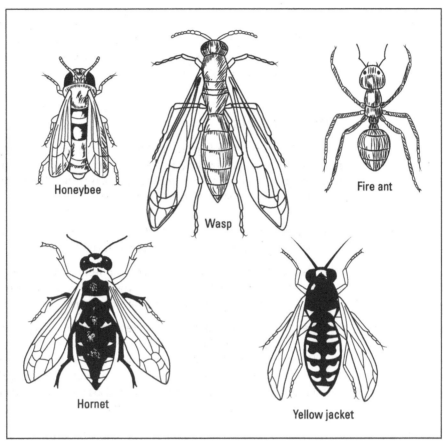

FIGURE 17-1: These five groups of insects are the ones whose venom most often triggers allergic insect string reactions in humans.

The following sections provide more details on the stinging *Hymenoptera* insects and how they can affect you.

Honeybees

Bees are the most important pollinators in the insect world, and they also make honey, one of the oldest crops harvested by humans. Honeybees are either domestic — raised in hives for commercial purposes — or wild. Wild honeybees usually build their hives, which may contain thousands of bees, in tree hollows or old logs. Here's more important information about these hard-working insects:

>> **Appearance:** They have hairy bodies with yellow and black markings.

>> **Habitat:** These insects are widespread throughout most of the United States. However, because honeybees prefer warmer climates, they tend to cause more problems in areas such as southern California, where they're one of the leading causes of insect sting reactions.

» **Behavior:** Honeybees aren't usually aggressive away from their hives. Female workers are the only honeybees that sting. They give their lives to protect their hives when they leave their large stingers in their victims — the only stinging insect that does this.

Yellow jackets

These ground-dwelling insects are the most frequent causes of stings in most of the United States, particularly in the northern states. Like paper wasps (see the next section), yellow jackets build paper nests, but they enclose them. Other important characteristics of yellow jackets are

» **Appearance:** Similar to hornets, they have bright yellow and black markings. Unlike hornets, they don't have a dark band under their eyes.

» **Habitat:** Yellow jackets usually build their nests in the ground, wall tunnels, crevices, and hollow logs. Therefore, you may encounter them more often while working in your yard, gardening, or farming.

» **Behavior:** Yellow jackets can be aggressive and may sting — sometimes repeatedly — with minimum provocation, especially if food is around. They like the taste of soft drinks and may dive right into the container. In fact many people get stung while drinking a beverage. Because female yellow jackets require protein in their diets, they many also go after meat (for example, hamburger at your cookout) as a food of choice.

Wasps

Watch for the so-called *paper wasps*, which get their name from the papier-mâché honeycomb nest that they build. These nests can be several inches in diameter, and the wasps often locate them in shrubs, under the eaves of houses and barns, and sometimes in pipes on playgrounds or under patio furniture. Here are other important points to keep in mind about wasps:

» **Appearance:** Wasps have hairless bodies with narrow waists and black or brown markings.

» **Habitat:** Wasps are primarily a problem in the southern United States.

» **Behavior:** Wasps are easy to provoke and can sting repeatedly and in large numbers when disturbed.

Most solitary wasps — except for velvet ants (also wasps, despite their name) — are much less aggressive and usually sting humans only if handled. Despite their bad reputation, farmers often consider wasps useful, because many of them feed on other insects that harm crops and trees.

Hornets

Related to yellow jackets and wasps, hornets build large papier-mâché nests several feet in diameter, which are often hard for humans to see, because hornets frequently nest in tree hollows or high in tree branches. In North America, the two varieties of this insect that concern people the most are white-faced hornets (also known as *bald-faced hornets*) and yellow hornets:

>> **Appearance:** Hornets are usually larger than other *Hymenoptera*, with short waists, compact black bodies, sparse hair, multiple yellow or white stripes, and a dark band under the eyes.

>> **Habitat:** Hornets often build their oval or pear-shaped nests in trees and shrubs. They're especially prevalent in the southern United States.

>> **Behavior:** Hornets are extremely aggressive, especially when close to their nests and, like wasps, can sting repeatedley.

Fire ants

Although you may think it's odd that these insects are included with buzzing, stinging insects, fossil evidence indicates that ants probably evolved from wasps. Count your blessings that out of the estimated one quadrillion ants living on this planet (even more numerous than *For Dummies* books), you only need to contend with four species of stinging fire ants in the United States, depending on where you live.

Of the fire ant species, two are native and two were inadvertently introduced from South America in the early decades of the 20th century. Here's what you need to know when dealing with these fierce insects:

>> **Appearance:** Fire ants are red or black and resemble typical, nonstinging ants, except they have a well-developed rear stinger. (If they've ever stung you, you know how well-developed that stinger is!)

>> **Habitat:** These ants are well established in the Gulf Coast U.S. states and Puerto Rico and are spreading to other southern states. They build large, hardened mounds several inches high and one to two feet wide, which are very common along sidewalks and roadways in the southeastern

United States. Because fire ant's nests are underground, getting rid of these creatures is extremely difficult.

» **Behavior:** These insects are very aggressive, especially if you disturb their mounds. They've developed a particularly effective way of inflicting damage: They anchor themselves to their victims with their powerful jaws and then pivot themselves (they're also quite limber) to deliver multiple stings, in a semicircular pattern, from their rear stinger. Fire ant stings usually produce pustules, sometimes within 24 hours. The most aggressive fire ants are the red imported fire ant, *Solenopsis invicta*. This species stings livestock, injures crops, and can cause short circuits by building mounds around electrical equipment.

THE BUZZ ON KILLER BEES

Killer bees, the infamous result of breeding between wild South American bees and African honeybees that were accidentally released in Brazil in 1956, have been grabbing a lot of headlines. More properly called *Africanized honeybees,* these hybrid bees have gradually migrated northward from South America, establishing themselves in many parts of Central America and entering southern Texas back in 1990.

Africanized honeybees are present in parts of Texas, Arizona, and California and are gradually spreading through other southern parts of the United States. They don't survive in colder climates, but occasionally forage into northern parts of the United States during the summer months. These bees are less selective in their hive sites than native honeybees — the descendants of European honeybees brought to the Americans from the Old World by colonists and immigrants over the last three centuries — and may nest in holes in outside walls, old tires, in the ground, around fence posts, and even in water meter vaults in front yards of some homes.

The venom of so-called killer bees isn't any different or more dangerous than most other wild or domestic native bees. Killer bees have a bad reputation primarily because of their aggressive behavior. When provoked, killer bees tend to attack in swarms, inflicting many more stings on their unfortunate targets than other types of bees do. If a swam of killer bees (or any other type of stinging insect) attacks you, drop face down on the ground, curl up, and protect your head as much as possible.

Scientists hope that killer bees will slowly migrate northwards and will breed with less aggressive homegrown honeybees, thus resulting in mellower and better-behaved subsequent generations, although this has yet to occur. The main damage that killer bees actually cause is economic, because they often interfere with the pollination of crops by domestic honeybees.

Diagnosing Your Stings

In addition to physically examining your sting reaction, taking a thorough medical history is the first step in properly diagnosing and managing insect hypersensitivity (as with any other allergic condition). Your physician needs to know whether you've been stung in the past and the symptoms you've experienced. Providing your physician with as much possible information about your current sting is also very important. These sections discuss how to identify what stinging insect may be causing your allergic reaction as well as the types of tests your physician may use to help diagnose your allergy.

Know your stinger

Figuring out which bug is bugging you may be a little easier if your physician knows all the circumstances about your sting. For example:

>> If you're clipping the hedges when you get stung, yellow jackets or hornets are the likely suspects.

>> A hornet may sting you while you're sitting under a tree or near a bush without obvious provocation.

>> Insects that sting your feet while you're walking outside barefoot or in sandals are most likely yellow jackets — they don't like being stepped on!

>> Getting stung while lounging on a patio chair may indicate that your chair harbors a wasp nest.

>> Stinging that occurs while you stop to smell the roses is usually the result of honeybees, which like to feed among flowers.

>> If you're stung while changing your tire on a rainy night in Georgia, you may be on top of a fire ant mound.

REMEMBER

To further identify the insect responsible for your reaction, try to provide your physician with the following information:

>> Your activities at the time you were stung

>> Where you were when you were stung

>> Where the insect stung you on your body

>> The types of insects that seem active in the area where you were stung

If you're able to capture the creature that stung you, bring it with you to your physician's office. Knowing exactly what stung you greatly helps your physician determine how to treat your reaction and hopefully may help you prevent further reactions. For example, if a honeybee stings you, you'll probably have a stinger and a dead bee as evidence.

Allergy skin testing

If you've had a serious, systemic reaction to an insect sting, your physician will usually recommend allergy skin or blood testing (see Chapter 4). This procedure can determine whether your reaction is the result of an allergic response. If it is, allergy testing can determine the specific cause of your reaction — you may be sensitive to more than one insect — and the extent of your sensitivity.

Because you may be at a higher risk of having a similar reaction in the future (due to increased sensitization from your previous insect sting), and considering that such reactions can be potentially dangerous, allergy skin or blood testing for insect sting hypersensitivity will help your physician to determine appropriate and effective prevention measures.

TECHNICAL STUFF

To determine whether you have one or more sensitivities to the various *Hymenoptera* insects, your physician will need to perform skin or blood tests to venom extracts from each of the stinging insects. The results can help them determine the advisability of initiating venom immunotherapy (VIT), which we explain in the section "Long-term treatment: Venom immunotherapy" later in this chapter. Allergen extracts for skin or blood testing and immunotherapy for the diagnosis and treatment of bites of *triatoma* and other biting insects aren't commercially available.

Preventing and Managing Reactions

Effectively managing your sensitivity to insect stings can mean the difference between enjoying the great outdoors relatively worry-free or risking recurrences of serious allergic reactions. Here we outline some strategies to help reduce your risk of experiencing a serious allergic reaction and how to administer the appropriate treatment if you do get stung.

Avoiding getting stung and more

The first step you can take to effectively manage your sensitivity to insect stings (and this is no great surprise!) is to avoid getting stung. An ounce of avoidance is worth a pound of medication.

TIP

If you have an insect sting hypersensitivity, we advise consulting your physician about taking preventative measures, such as the following:

>> Avoid bugging insects, and they usually won't bug you. If stinging insects are in your vicinity, don't provoke them, but move quickly and calmly out of the area as possible. If you run, flap your arms, or otherwise get agitated, the insect may sting in self-defense. In general, avoid jerky, fast movements because these can startle and provoke insect stings.

>> Make sure that your children don't poke, hit, or otherwise play with insect hives, nests, or mounds.

>> Hire a trained extermination professional to check your home and its surroundings for insect nests. (We don't advise doing this home improvement project yourself.)

>> Stay away from strongly scented lotions, perfumes, colognes, and hair products. Likewise, don't wear brightly colored or flower-print clothing. Try khaki and other light-colored apparel. Also, avoid loose clothing that may trap insects.

>> Don't use electric hedge clippers and power mowers. For some reason, electricity really excites *Hymenoptera* insects, and you don't want to be part of their excitement. In general, we advise against doing yardwork yourself if you have a stinging insect hypersensitivity.

>> If you work outdoors, cover up from head to toe with long pants, a long-sleeved shirt, socks, closed shoes, a hat, and work gloves. Wear closed shoes (not sandals) or sneakers when you're outdoors, and don't go out in your stocking feet or barefoot.

>> Practice caution near flowery plants, blooming orchards (they're in bloom because something's busy pollinating them), bushes, clover fields, eaves, attics, garbage containers, and picnic areas.

>> Have insecticides at hand to zap stinging insects before they zap you (insect repellents don't work on stinging insects). Bear in mind that if these products kill insects, then they're also not too good for you either. Therefore, make sure you use insecticides properly as per the manufacturer's instructions to limit your exposure to the toxins.

>> Be careful when eating or drinking outdoors or when you're near areas where food and beverages are served. Also, cover the opening to your beverage and never drink from a container that's been left outdoors.

>> Check to see whether the insect left a stinger, which usually looks like a black thorn or splinter, in your skin. Carefully remove the stinger, using a tweezer to pry or a credit card to flick or scrape the stinger from your skin (certainly the least expensive way to use a credit card!). Never squeeze the stinger with your

fingers in an effort to remove it from your skin. Doing so pumps more venom into your body, making your reaction worse.

>> After a sting, walk slowly, don't run. Running may increase your body's absorption of the venom. (See the next section for more important tips on treating stings.)

Treating local reactions

You can manage the symptoms of local reactions (itching, swelling, and pain) until they pass with simple remedies, such as:

>> **Cold compresses,** which can help reduce local pain and swelling

>> **Local anesthetic cream, oral antihistamines, and oral analgesics,** which may help relieve the pain and itching of skin reactions

Treating systemic reactions

Hives and angioedema (deep swellings) can sometimes be the first signs of an impending anaphylactic insect sting reaction. Because it's impossible to predict whether these systemic symptoms will or will not progress to anaphylaxis, it's therefore safe to immediately administer epinephrine (see the next section) than to wait until the reaction becomes life-threatening.

If the systemic reaction is limited to hives and angioedema, then your best strategy is to avoid further aggravating your skin while soothing it as much as possible. Advisable steps include

>> Bathing and washing with lukewarm water and using gentle soaps instead of harsh ones to reduce itching. Hot baths and showers may intensify your symptoms. Likewise, avoid hot environments and keep your home — especially your bedroom — cool.

>> Patting yourself dry with a soft towel after bathing and applying moisturizers immediately afterward to seal in moisture.

>> Wearing comfortable, loose, cotton clothing instead of tight-fitting garments.

>> Taking oral antihistamines may also be advisable to help relieve your symptoms.

Treating urgent insect sting cases

If you're prone to serious systemic insect sting reactions and you get stung despite taking protective measures, be prepared to prevent a life-threatening reaction (anaphylaxis). Consult with your physician about getting a prescription for an injectable epinephrine kit (such as EpiPen or Auvi-Q), which contains an injectable dose of epinephrine.

A new single dose epinephrine nasal spray called "neffy" has recently become available and may be an alternative to the injectable form of treatment for patients who weigh more than 66 pounds. Discuss this alternative with your physician as a possible approach to treating a severe allergic reaction. For more information on neffy turn to Chapter 14.

WARNING

Make sure your physician shows you how to use the injectable epinephrine. Learning the proper technique for administering epinephrine in your physician's office is much better than trying to figure it out for the first time when you're having a reaction.

TIP

Keep these important points about using an epinephrine kit in mind:

>> Having more than one injectable epinephrine is a good idea. You may want to keep more than one injector with you when traveling or going on an extended outing because the initial injection wears off in 30 minutes and you may need another one before you can get to emergency care.

>> Store any epinephrine injectors you're not keeping with you at room temperature and protect them from sunlight.

>> If your child is at risk for anaphylactic reactions to insect stings, you should consider keeping one injector at their school or daycare (in consultation with the personnel at these places). Make sure personnel at those locations know how and when to administer this medication.

>> Many people also keep an antihistamine such as diphenhydramine (Benadryl) with them in case of a serious insect sting reaction. However, we advise you not to rely solely on an antihistamine, which can take up to 30 minutes to start becoming effective. In addition, this medication won't prevent anaphylaxis. Administration of epinephrine should be the initial treatment for anaphylaxis prior to the use of any antihistamine.

WARNING

>> Remember that you need to get emergency treatment immediately after administration of epinephrine, because the drug's effect usually doesn't last more than 30 minutes.

>> If you're at risk for anaphylaxis, we advise you to wear a MedicAlert bracelet or necklace in case you're unable to speak during a reaction.

Long-term treatment: Venom immunotherapy

If you've had a serious systemic reaction to an insect sting, your physician will probably advise you to consider *venom immunotherapy* (VIT). This form of immunotherapy (allergy shots) is effective in about 98 percent of cases.

TECHNICAL STUFF

VIT injections are usually initially administered on a weekly basis beginning with an extremely small dose of venom from the insect to which you react. Physician initiate a rapid *desensitization* process so that you reach a maintenance dose as soon and as safely as possible. After you've worked up to a *maintenance dose*, shots are usually given every four weeks during the first year and every six to eight weeks in subsequent years.

After three to five years of VIT, depending on the degree of your sensitivity and the level of your initial allergic episode, your physician may recommend that you discontinue immunotherapy if skin or blood tests are negative or the venom-specific IgE antibodies in your system have dropped to an insignificant level. Most experts agree that at the end of five years, VIT can usually be safely discontinued. For the vast majority of patients who have completed a course of VIT, the threat of another life-threatening reaction to an insect sting is remote.

6

The Part of Tens

Chapter **18**

Top Ten List of Allergy Triggers

You live in a world surrounded by potential allergy triggers. These allergens cause various clinical symptoms associated with many different areas of the body. These allergens include the following:

REMEMBER

» Pollens

» Animal danders

» Dust mites

» Mold spores

» Certain foods

» Some medications

» Venom from stinging insects

Allergens can cause a wide variety of medical conditions for millions of people around the world. These medical conditions can present as a minor annoyance, such as a runny nose; as a serious medical problem — for example, asthma — or even anaphylaxis, which is a potentially life-threatening reaction (see Chapter 14 for more information on this topic).

In most cases, under proper medical supervision, physicians such as allergy specialists can accurately identify the allergic triggers involved in the clinical reaction and initiate effective treatment to manage your condition. In this chapter, we showcase the top ten list of allergy triggers.

DOCTOR SAYS

Thanks to medical research in the field of allergy and immunology, our understanding of the underlying allergic triggers involved in clinical reactions has allowed physicians to properly diagnose and identify the cause of allergic symptoms. In addition, this has led to the development of appropriate and effective treatment plans for managing your condition.

More than likely in the coming years even greater success will be achieved in preventing and treating allergic diseases, and patients everywhere will be the direct beneficiaries of these significant medical advances.

Pollens

Pollens are universal features of life on Earth. Plants that depend on wind rather than insects for pollination, such as some types of grasses, trees, and weeds produce pollens that are released into the air at specific times of the year. They can often end up in the eyes, nose, throat, and lungs, causing reactions in individuals with allergies.

Pollen Food Allergy Syndrome (PFAS), also called Oral Allergy Syndrome (OAS), is linked to seasonal pollen allergies and can mimic an allergic reaction to the food; however, symptoms tend to be mild, transient, and restricted to the oral cavity.

TIP

Avoid eating these raw foods especially during pollen allergy season (trees in spring, ragweed in the fall), because frequently OAS worsens during the particular pollen season. Sometimes baking the food or peeling it before eating (for example, apples) can reduce the cross-reaction of the food because high temperatures break down the proteins associated with OAS, and in some cases those allergenic proteins can be concentrated on the skin of the fruit.

REMEMBER

Often referred to as hay fever, *allergic rhinitis* triggered by pollens is the most common allergic disease in the United States. Classic symptoms of this condition include

>> Runny, stuffy nose

>> Sneezing

>> Itchy, watery eyes

Pollens can also trigger allergic asthma symptoms in susceptible individuals. You can find more discussion of pollens in Chapter 4.

Molds

Airborne mold spores occur almost everywhere on the planet (you might still be safe from mold at the North and South poles). Outdoor molds are present throughout the year, but peak levels occur during the summer months. Those outdoor molds usually grow on field crops such as corn and wheat and are also found on decaying matter such as compost, hay, and piles of leaves.

Indoor molds can be found in crawl spaces in homes and in damp, dark areas such as inside walls around pipes. They particularly grow in damp places within the home such as bathrooms, basements, leaks around windows, ceiling tiles, drywall, or carpet, especially where there has been flooding.

REMEMBER

Molds can trigger symptoms similar to those caused by pollens, such as red, itchy watery eyes, stuffy or runny nose, or even coughing or wheezing.

For more moldy matters, turn to Chapter 4.

Dust Mites

Although you have probably never seen them, dust mites produce waste (fecal matter) that is the most prevalent form of house dust allergen. These tiny creatures thrive in dark and humid environments such as mattresses, pillows, and box springs. Dust mites also survive in blankets, carpets, towels, and drapery.

TIP

Covering pillows, mattresses, and box springs in allergen-proof encasings can help to control dust mites. It's also highly advisable to wash all linens in hot water (at least 130 degrees) every one to two weeks. If possible, remove carpeting and thick rugs, replacing them with hard wood, linoleum, or tile floors, which are much easier to keep clean.

To find out more about dust mites, see Chapter 4.

Animal Danders

Dander from animals is a significant source of allergy triggers for many people with allergies. These skin flakes are produced by all warm-blooded household pets regardless of their hair length. The protein in their dander (and saliva) can trigger allergic symptoms in their owners and other susceptible individuals who might be exposed to the dander, such as coughing, wheezing, and nasal congestion. Interestingly, cat allergen causes more sudden and severe symptoms than dog allergens, because cat allergen is smaller, lighter and stickier than dog allergens. As a result, feline proteins linger longer in the air and cling more easily to furniture and fabrics.

TIP

Keeping your pet outdoors whenever possible, or at least out of the bedroom, can help control exposure to animal dander. Always wash your hands and the hands of anyone else who touches the pet and try to wash the animal with water at least once per week. Doing so will help to reduce the amount of dander that can circulate within the home.

For deeper dander details, you can turn to Chapter 5.

Foods

Your immune system has the ability to develop specific IgE antibodies against a number of food allergens (see Chapter 2 for a discussion of IgE antibodies). This can result in a range of adverse food allergic reactions, including nasal, respiratory, skin, gastrointestinal, and oral symptoms occurring separately or in combinations.

WARNING

The most extreme of all allergic food symptoms is referred to as anaphylaxis, affecting several body organs simultaneously, and even becoming life-threatening (see Chapter 14 for more information on this topic).

SEE YOUR
DOCTOR

Allergy tests in combination with a good history of food reaction help to make the diagnosis. This may include undergoing a double-blind placebo — controlled oral food challenge where neither you, nor your physician know the contents of the test. This type of test should be done under close medical supervision (see Chapter 15 for details on this test and other types of food allergy testing).

REMEMBER

The most common food allergens are

>> Peanuts

>> Shellfish

>> Fish

>> Tree nuts

>> Eggs

>> Cow's milk

>> Wheat

>> Soy

>> Sesame

If you're hungering for more information on food allergy, turn to Chapter 14.

Medications

Drug allergies can occur with certain drugs in people who have developed allergic sensitivities to one of the otherwise harmless components of these drugs. As a result, your immune system produces IgE antibodies in response to these allergens and can, upon re-exposure, cause allergic clinical symptoms. Many factors can determine the risk of a reaction including the dosage level, the route of administration (orally versus injection), and how long you've taken the drug.

The most frequent type of adverse reactions to medications occurs with penicillin and its related compounds (such as amoxicillin). Other drugs that can cause allergic reactions include cephalosporins, sulfonamides, and insulin.

TIP

Determining the source of the drug reaction can be difficult if you are taking more than one medication. Keeping a symptom diary can help to identify the likeliest cause of the adverse reaction.

For more information on adverse drug reactions, see Chapter 16.

Insect Stings

Many insects can bite or sting, but only a small percentage of stinging insects can produce venom that can trigger an allergic reaction. The five groups that cause the majority of reactions, all members of the *Hymenoptera* order, are

- » Honeybees
- » Yellowjackets
- » Wasps
- » Hornets
- » Fire ants

REMEMBER

Insect stings can cause small local reactions (redness, itching, swelling, and pain at the sting site), large local reactions (extreme swelling that extends from the sting site), systemic reactions (hives and swelling over a large area of the body), and even life-threatening reactions (anaphylactic symptoms such as swelling of the tongue and throat).

TIP

The first step to manage sensitivity to insect sings is to avoid getting stung! Some common tips are to stay away from strongly scented lotions, perfumes, and colognes. Limit eating or drinking outdoors and avoid areas where *al fresco* food and beverages are being served. Be cautious around flowery plants, eaves, attic, garbage containers, and picnic areas.

SEE YOUR DOCTOR

If you're at risk of serious systemic reactions to insect stings, consult your physician about getting a prescription for an injectable epinephrine kit (such as EpiPen or Auvi-Q), which contains an injectable dose of epinephrine. A new form of nasal epinephrine spray, called "neffy" has recently been FDA approved. Consult your physician for more information.

If you're buzzing for more information on insect stings, see Chapter 17.

Latex

Allergic contact dermatitis is a condition that occurs when the skin physically contacts an allergen causing a reaction at the site of exposure. The resulting inflammation leads to a skin rash, blistering, itching, and a burning sensation. This usually occurs 36 to 48 hours following exposure to the allergen.

REMEMBER

Thousands of chemicals in use today can potentially trigger allergic contact dermatitis. Millions of Americans experience sensitivity to latex, derived from the sap of the Brazilian rubber tree. Common latex and synthetic rubber containing items include

>> Rubber bands

>> Erasers

>> Rubber handgrips on bicycles and golf clubs

>> Balloons and rubber toys

>> Medical products such as surgical gloves and adhesive bandages

TIP

Most of these products have non-latex alternatives. Patch testing is available to confirm if natural rubber is actually triggering your dermatitis.

To find out more about latex reactions and allergic contact dermatitis, see Chapter 12.

Nickel

Allergy to nickel, a metallic element found in many of the objects that you touch daily, can produce an eczema-type rash, itching, and hive-like eruptions. This sort of sensitivity is much more common in women, possibly because women tend to wear more costume jewelry than men, starting at an earlier age. Men commonly experience allergy to nickel due to an occupational allergic contact dermatitis resulting from working in areas such as mining and construction.

TIP

One approach to controlling nickel allergy is to wear only jewelry with higher gold content and less nickel. Another preventive measure it to wear a protective layer between your skin and items that contain nickel. You may also want to carry a pouch or other type of enclosure with you that holds your keys, watch, coins, and other metal objects. Perspiration can leach nickel out of these objects, allowing the skin to absorb the element and trigger an allergic rash. This response commonly occurs on the wrist under a metal watch.

For a deeper dive into this element, see Chapter 12.

Poison Ivy, Poison Oak, Poison Sumac

The leaves of these poison plants, native to most parts of North America, contain *urushiol*, an oily resin (oleoresin) that can cause blisters and a streaky red rash on skin areas brushed by the plant.

It usually takes a second contact with urushiol for symptoms to appear, typically within two days, and then spread to new areas of the body for several days after the initial outbreak. The majority of contacts result from direct exposure of bare skin to these plants while camping or hiking.

TIP

The easiest way to prevent exposure to these allergens is to avoid all contact with poison plants. The best way to do so is to recognize their characteristic three leaf cluster (*"leaves of three, let them be"*). We also advise to wear clothing that covers as much of your skin as possible and wash off any part of your skin that you may have exposed.

SEE YOUR
DOCTOR

If you nonetheless experience a too-close encounter with a poison plant and a resulting rash becomes widespread, see your doctor for further treatment.

To read more about poison plants, turn to Chapter 12.

Chapter **19**

Top Ten Body Organs Affected by Allergies

Allergies, including asthma, *atopic dermatitis* (eczema), *allergic rhinitis* (hay fever), food allergies, and pollen food allergy syndrome (PFAS), can cause symptoms in a multitude of different ways, depending on which organ of the body is being affected. Your symptoms may vary widely from mild (such as a runny nose or itchy eyes) to very severe and may even be life-threatening (*anaphylaxis*). You may also notice that your symptoms are worse at certain times of the year, particularly if you suffer from allergic rhinitis or asthma.

REMEMBER

In this chapter we discuss how allergies can affect various organs throughout the body and what symptoms you may experience. Being able to recognize your symptoms and identify certain triggers is important in helping your physician accurately diagnose and treat your individual allergic condition.

Eyes

Allergies often manifest in the eyes as allergic conjunctivitis. This condition makes the eyes swollen, red, itchy, and watery, causing significant discomfort and sometimes blurred vision. This ailment often coexists with allergic rhinitis and, in most cases, the same allergens involved with that condition can trigger seasonal or perennial (all year long) outbreaks of allergic conjunctivitis.

REMEMBER

The three basic approaches to treating most allergic diseases in general also apply to managing allergic conjunctivitis. They are as follows:

>> **Avoidance:** Eliminating or at least lessening your exposure to allergens and irritants, which can often result in less severe symptoms and decreased need for medications (see Chapter 5 for a full discussion on allergen avoidance).

>> **Medication:** Your physician may prescribe one or more types of medications, including eyedrops to help manage your condition (see Chapter 6 for information on medications).

>> **Immunotherapy:** If avoidance and medications don't provide effective relief, you might want to consult with an allergist to consider immunotherapy (allergy shots) for your condition (see Chapter 4 for details on allergy shots).

Ears

Allergies can increase susceptibility to middle ear infections (*otitis media*). The connection between allergies and these infections is due to inflammation of the Eustachian tubes, which can lead to fluid buildup and infection within the ears.

REMEMBER

The middle ear is the part of the organ that's affected most by inflammatory disease processes with the resulting infections specially common in young children and infants. In fact, otitis media is the most common reason in the United States for pediatric sick visits and can adversely affect the learning ability of children due to potential hearing loss.

In many cases allergic rhinitis (hay fever) precedes an ear infection. Other conditions can also increase the chances of developing ear infections. These conditions include the ones listed here, which can all lead to frequent nasal congestion:

>> Sinusitis (from exposure to allergens, pollutants, and other environmental irritants)

>> Enlarged adenoids

>> Unrepaired cleft palate

>> Nasal polyps

>> Hypothyroidism

SEE YOUR DOCTOR

The most important step in diagnosing a suspected ear infection involves examination with an otoscope to look for signs of infection. Treatment usually includes a course of antibiotic.

For an earful on ear infections, refer to Chapter 7.

Nose

Allergic rhinitis is one of the classic allergy symptoms. This condition often leads to the following nasal issues that negatively impact quality of life:

>> Runny nose

>> Sneezing

>> Congestion

>> Post-nasal drip

Allergists distinguish between the different forms of allergic rhinitis, which are classified according to the various types and patterns of exposure. These forms include

>> Seasonal allergic rhinitis

>> Perennial allergic rhinitis

>> Occupational allergic rhinitis

REMEMBER

Studies have shown that 80 percent of people with allergic rhinitis develop this condition before their 20th birthday. Anyone who experiences significant nasal symptoms should consult a physician to determine whether these symptoms are the result of allergic rhinitis, nonallergic rhinitis, a sinus infection, or part of a respiratory problem.

SEE YOUR DOCTOR

Many allergy sufferers mistakenly assume that they're experiencing a lingering cold that affects them every spring or whenever the weather changes. Even though viral infections such as the common cold and various strains of influenza (flu) follow cyclical patterns, the frequency of these illnesses usually isn't as consistent or as constant as allergic rhinitis. That's why a proper diagnosis is critical for the effective and appropriate management of these medical conditions.

To discover more about your nose's woes, see Chapter 6.

Sinus

Sinus inflammation, or *sinusitis,* is frequently associated with allergies. Swollen nasal passages can block the sinuses, leading to pressure, headaches, and sometimes infection.

REMEMBER

The sinuses that surround your nose are referred to as *paranasal sinuses,* which are hollow cavities in the bones that surround your nasal cavity. The three types of paranasal sinuses come in pairs, one on each side of the nose, and are named for the bones that house them:

>> **Maxillary:** The largest sinuses located in your cheekbones.

>> **Frontal:** The sinuses that reside in your forehead above your eyes.

>> **Ethmoid:** The sinuses found immediately behind your eyes and nose.

>> **Sphenoid:** Located behind the nose between the eyes in the center of the cranial base, it's lined with cells that make mucus and keep the nose from drying out.

TECHNICAL STUFF

Sinuses are a vital part of your body's defense against airborne bacteria, viruses, irritants, and allergens that you constantly inhale. Under normal circumstances, the mucus in your sinuses traps most of these invaders, and the *cilia* — the tiny hairlike projections of certain cells that line the sinuses — sweep the mucus and potential threats to your immune system into the nasal passages, draining them into your throat, and from there, eliminating them through the digestive system. With rhinitis, the nasal and sinus linings swell, narrowing the sinus drainage openings and retaining mucus which then becomes infected, leading to sinusitis. In some cases, mainly in adults, the sinuses themselves are diseased, and because of the primary disease within the sinus cavities, they're more susceptible to infection.

For more sinus science, refer to Chapter 7.

Throat

Allergies can irritate the back of the throat, causing *pharyngitis.* The symptoms of this condition include

>> Sore, scratchy throat that can make swallowing difficult and painful

>> Runny nose

>> Cough

>> Headache

>> Hoarse voice

REMEMBER

Patients with pharyngitis can present with swollen lymph nodes and a fever that lasts several days. These patients can also suffer from concurrent sinusitis and acute otitis media. Many of these pharyngitis cases are caused by a viral or bacterial infection in addition to irritants, smoke, and allergies.

In contrast to pharyngitis, *laryngitis* is an inflammation of the voice box, otherwise known as the larynx, located at the top of the neck. This part of the throat controls breathing, swallowing, and the ability to speak. As opposed to pharyngitis, individuals with laryngitis lose their voice for as long as the vocal cords are inflamed. Laryngitis can occur from the following:

>> Infections

>> Allergies

>> Overuse of the vocal cords

>> Gastroesophageal reflux disease (GERD)

SEE YOUR DOCTOR

Make sure a physician properly diagnoses you to differentiate between pharyngitis and laryngitis so you receive the appropriate medical therapy.

To find out more about allergies and your throat, see Chapter 4.

Esophagus

Your food pipe or food tube is known in the medical field as your *esophagus*. Ingested food passes from the mouth, through the pharynx, and then the esophagus, emptying into the upper part of the stomach. In most adults the esophagus is about 10 inches long and has two muscular rings, known as sphincters, found both at the top and the bottom of the esophagus. The lower sphincter is essential in preventing reflux of acidic stomach content and protecting the lining of the esophagus.

Inflammation of the esophagus is known as *esophagitis*, which can cause painful swallowing and is often managed by controlling reflux and treating any potential inflammation or infection.

TECHNICAL STUFF

The normal esophagus does not contain any eosinophils. But in eosinophilic Esophagitis (EOE) the eosinophil is a dominant cell in this organ. Eosinophilic esophagitis (EOE) is known to be an allergic condition of the esophagus and is increasingly viewed as a major cause of scarring, narrowing, and swallowing difficulties, known as *dysphagia*, for both children and adults. A type of white blood cell, called an *eosinophil*, builds up in the lining in the esophagus and can inflame or injure the esophageal lining, leading to dysphagia.

REMEMBER

EOE can be triggered by food allergy, acid reflux, or even seasonal allergies. Treatment options include elimination diets (see Chapter 15), topical steroids, acid suppressors, and monoclonal antibodies (see Chapter 6 for medication information).

Lungs

For individuals with asthma, allergies are a common and significant trigger. Inflammation of the airways is the most important underlying factor in asthma. Allergens can irritate sensitive airways of the lungs, leading to these characteristic symptoms:

>> Wheezing

>> Shortness of breath

>> Coughing

>> Chest tightness

In many cases, asthma is due to *atopy*, which is the tendency to develop hypersensitivity to allergens. However, a significant number of people with asthma, especially adults, don't have a history of allergies. In addition, many people with asthma also suffer from rhinitis, both in its allergic and nonallergic forms.

The airways of the lungs are vital to your health. This network of bronchial tubes enables your lungs to absorb oxygen into the bloodstream and eliminate carbon dioxide in a process known as *respiration*, or breathing.

SEE YOUR DOCTOR

Most individuals take breathing for granted, and you usually don't think about until something interferes with this process by obstructing your airways, which is what happens in uncontrolled asthma. That's why controlling your allergies is a vital part of asthma therapy.

To breathe easier about lung health and effective asthma management, see Chapter 10.

Stomach

Food allergies can represent a distinct immediate IgE-mediated or delayed cell-mediated hypersensitivity reaction within the gastrointestinal tract (refer to Chapter 2 for the role IgE and cell-mediated reactions plays in allergic conditions). Symptoms range from mild discomfort like nausea, cramping, and upset stomach to vomiting, diarrhea, and potentially severe allergic reactions in the case of anaphylaxis (check out Chapter 14).

REMEMBER

Allergic reactions involving the digestive system can develop within a few minutes to several hours after ingesting food allergens. This means that identifying the exact food allergen culprit may be difficult.

Gastrointestinal food allergic reactions generally are accompanied by other atopic conditions including allergic rhinitis and *atopic dermatitis* (eczema). The major food allergens that have been identified are mainly proteins found in specific foods, including:

» Peanuts

» Shellfish

» Fish

» Tree nuts

» Eggs

» Cow's milk

» Wheat

» Soy

» Sesame

SEE YOUR DOCTOR

If your physician can't clearly identify the cause of the gastrointestinal reaction, then skin or blood testing may be recommended. Oral food challenges, which involve ingesting under medical supervision very small quantities of food that may contain suspected allergens, may be undertaken as an additional step to make an accurate diagnosis of food allergy.

To get your fill on managing food allergies, see Chapter 15.

Skin

Allergies are a major culprit behind various skin conditions. Atopic dermatitis and contact dermatitis are types of allergic eczema, causing itchy, red, and inflamed patches on the skin. Atopic dermatitis is more than just dry itchy skin, however. It has a significant adverse effect on your quality of life and can lead to complications such as bacterial and viral skin infections.

REMEMBER

Atopic dermatitis frequently occurs in conjunction with allergic respiratory diseases such as allergic rhinitis and asthma, often preceding other allergic symptoms. The hallmark of this disease is the vicious cycle of significant itching due to the inflammation causing dry skin, leading to constant scratching. This results in more irritation and inflammation and damaged skin. That's why controlling the itching is a key element of successfully treating this condition.

SEE YOUR DOCTOR

Contact dermatitis is a condition that occurs when the skin physically contacts an allergen that triggers a reaction, usually at the site of exposure. The reaction often produces inflammation resulting in symptoms such as a skin rash, blistering, itching, and burning sensations with cracked or crusting areas of the skin. This immunologic reaction typically appears 36 to 48 hours following exposure to the allergen, caused frequently by the resin of poison ivy, latex, and nickel. Patch testing is usually performed to identify the offending allergen.

To get the skinny about dermatitis, see Chapter 12.

Lips and Tongue

Allergies sometimes lead to *angioedema*, a condition marked by rapid swelling of the deeper layers of the skin. This type of inflammation can be concerning when it affects the lips and tongue, potentially hindering breathing. Also known as *deep swellings*, this condition results in deeper tissue inflammation as compared to hives, which are seen mainly on the skin surface.

The swelling of angioedema is less likely to produce painful and burning sensations because angioedema occurs in deeper skin layers where fewer mast cells and sensory nerve endings reside. As a result, the lesions cause little or no itching.

REMEMBER

Angioedema affects the lips, tongue, and eyelids more frequently because these parts of your body have thinner skin and more blood circulation closer to the surface. That's why inflammation from angioedema can cause discomfort and temporary facial swelling. Angioedema often coexists with *urticaria* (hives), but the two conditions can occur independently.

For a fuller discussion of angioedema, head to Chapter 13.

Anaphylaxis: Many Organs Simultaneously

REMEMBER

As we note in this chapter's introduction and throughout this book, the most severe allergic reaction affecting the body's organs is anaphylaxis. This systemic and potentially life-threatening reaction impacts multiple organ systems simultaneously, causing symptoms such as

>> Widespread hives and itching over the body (*urticaria*)

>> Flushing, wheezing, and difficulty breathing

>> Low blood pressure (*hypotension*)

>> Nausea, vomiting, abdominal pain, and/or diarrhea

WARNING

These symptoms can progress to anaphylactic shock and loss of consciousness. Anaphylaxis requires urgent medical intervention with epinephrine to reverse its progression.

In the United States the most frequent causes of anaphylaxis are

>> Extreme allergic reactions to venom from stinging insects (*Hymenoptera*) such as honeybees, yellow jackets, hornets, and wasps (refer to Chapter 17)

>> Drugs such as penicillin and related compounds (see Chapter 16)

>> Foods, particularly peanuts and shellfish (see Chapter 15)

SEE YOUR DOCTOR

If you're at risk for anaphylaxis, be prepared to take the appropriate measures to quickly treat these life-threatening reactions. Have your physician prescribe an epinephrine injector and make sure you know how to use it so that in an emergency, epinephrine can be immediately administered.

Recently, the U.S. Food and Drug Administration approved the first non-injectable emergency treatment for allergic reactions, including life-threatening anaphylaxis, in the form of a single dose epinephrine nasal spray 2 mg called neffy. See Chapter 14 for more information on neffy and anaphylaxis.

Index

F

forced expiratory flow between 25 and 75 percent (FEF 25–75 percent), 151

forced expiratory volume (FEV1), 151

forced vital capacity (FVC), 151

formalin, 217

Formicidae family
  defined, 294
  fire ants, 297–298

FPIES (food protein-induced enterocolitis syndrome), 261

Franklin, Benjamin, 72, 173–174

frontal sinuses, 118–119

functional endoscopic sinus surgery, 124

FVC (forced vital capacity), 151

G

gammaglobulin, 26

gastroesophageal reflux disease (GERD), 170–172

gastrointestinal (GI) allergies, 256–257, 321. *See also* food allergies/hypersensitivities

gastrointestinal food hypersensitivity reactions, 256

gatekeepers, 54

generalized heat urticaria, 236–237

generalized urticaria, 258

genetic predisposition. *See* atopy

GERD (gastroesophageal reflux disease), 170–172

glaucoma, 169

gliadin, 261

grapefruit juice, 263

"grass grief," 59

grass pollens, 63, 87

gustatory rhinitis, 68–69

H

HAE (hereditary angioedema), 240–241

Haegarda (C1 esterase inhibitors), 241

hay fever. *See* allergic rhinitis

health equity, 142–143

health maintenance organizations (HMOs), 53–55

Healthy People 2020, 142

Heating, ventilation, and air-conditioning (HVAC) systems, 77

hereditary angioedema (HAE), 240–241

High Efficiency Particulate Air (HEPA) filters, 77, 165–166

histamines, 12–13, 34–35, 95

HIV/AIDS, 29, 117, 197

hives. *See* urticaria

HMOs (health maintenance organizations), 53–55

honeybees, 295–296

hormonal rhinitis, 68–69

hornets, 297

household triggers, 164

humanized monoclonal antibody, 206–207

humoral immunity, 28

humoral immunity (antibody response), 211–212

HVAC (Heating, ventilation, and air-conditioning) systems, 77

hydroxyzine (Atarax), 216

Hymenoptera insects, 311
  Apidae family
    defined, 294
    honeybees, 295–296
  Formicidae family
    defined, 294
    fire ants, 297–298
  Vespidae family
    defined, 294
    hornets, 297
    wasps, 296–297
    yellow jackets, 296

hyperresponsivity, 37–38

hypersensitivities, 8–9. *See also* food allergies/hypersensitivities

hyperthyroidism, 33, 169

hyposensitization, 73

hypothyroidism, 51

I

ibuprofen (Advil, Motrin), 232

icatibant injection (Firazyr), 241

ichthyosis, 196

idiopathic chronic nonallergic rhinitis, 68–69

idiosyncratic drug reactions, 20, 280

IgA antibodies, 26

IgD antibodies, 26

IgE antibodies (reaginic antibodies), 12, 26–28

systemic reactions, 293
treating
  life-threatening reactions, 303
  local reactions, 302
  systemic reactions, 302
  venom immunotherapy, 304
triatoma genus, 294
triggers, 293–298
urticaria and angioedema, 17, 235
insurance, 53–55
intolerance reactions, 239
intracutaneous tests, 271
IOS (impulse oscillometry), 151–152
ipratropium bromide, 110
irritant contact dermatitis, 210, 223. *See also* contact dermatitis
irritants
  allergic rhinitis, 65
  household, 81
itch-scratch cycle, 15, 194

J

JAK inhibitors, 207
jogger's nose, 110

K

Kalbitor (ecallantide), 241
ketoprofen (Actron, Orudis), 232
ketorolac (Acular), 112
ketotifen (Zaditor OTC), 112
Kids With Food Allergies, 146–147
killer bees (Africanized honeybees), 298
known side effects, 278

L

lactose intolerance, 262
lanadelumab-flyo (Takhzyro), 241
laryngeal edema, 258
laryngitis, 319
larynx, 152
latex, 167–168, 213–214, 312
less-common allergens, 254

leukotriene modifiers, 111
leukotrienes, 34–35
levocabastine (Livostin), 111
levocetirizine, 99
life-threatening reactions, insect stings
  defined, 293
  treating, 303
Livostin (levocabastine), 111
local reactions, insect stings
  large, local reactions, 293
  small, local reactions, 292
  treating, 302
lodoxamide (Alomide), 112
Lone Star Tick, 235
loratadine, 99
lymph nodes, 27
lymphoid tissues, 27

M

macrophages (scavenger cells), 29
malabsorption syndrome, 261
malocclusion, 70
managed care plans, 54–55
MAO inhibitors, 263
mast cells, 12, 26, 95, 268
  IgE-mediated reactions, 33–34
  mast cell stabilizers, 112
maxillary sinuses, 118–119
maximum midexpiratory flow (MMEF), 151
MedicAlert bracelets and pendants, 169, 260, 289
Medicare, 53
medication records, 286–287
medications. *See* drug allergies/hypersensitivities
meningitis, 119
mepyramine (Pyrilamine), 216
metabolic food reactions, 262–263
middle ear, 127–128
milk, 253, 256, 262
MMEF (maximum midexpiratory flow), 151
mold, 85–86, 163, 309
mometasone, 107
monosodium glutamate (MSG), 263–264
montelukast (Singulair), 111

Motrin (ibuprofen), 232

mouth breathing, 67

mupirocin nasal ointment, 123

Musk ambrette, 218

Mycolog Cream, 216

MyPurMist Handheld Vaporizer and Humidifier, 123

myringotomy, 130

N

naphazoline, 102

naproxen (Aleve), 232

NARES (nonallergic rhinitis with eosinophilia syndrome), 68–69

nasal corticosteroids, 105–107

nasal crease, 67

nasal decongestants, 102–103

nasal lavage, 123

nasal polyps, 131

nasal rebound (rhinitis medicamentosa), 61–62, 103, 117

nasal septum, 117

nasal smear, 50

nasal sprays, 62

  antihistamines, 100–101

  combination, 107–108

  cromolyn sodium, 109

  epinephrine nasal spray, 303

  ipratropium bromide, 110

  nasal corticosteroids, 105–107

nasal voice, 61

nasopharynx, 127–128

National Institutes of Health (NIH), 177, 179

natural rubber latex (NRL), 214

nedocromil sodium (Alocril), 112

neffy (epinephrine nasal spray), 260, 289, 303

New England Journal of Medicine, 54

nickel, 215, 313

nighttime (nocturnal) asthma, 160–161

NIH (National Institutes of Health), 177, 179

nitrites, 255

nocturnal (nighttime) asthma, 160–161

NOML (Not One More Life), 143

nonallergic (nonatopic) asthma, 144

nonallergic contact urticaria, 219, 239

nonallergic food hypersensitivities (non-IgE food reactions), 252, 261–262

nonallergic rhinitis, 68–69

nonallergic rhinitis with eosinophilia syndrome (NARES), 68–69

nonatopic (nonallergic) asthma, 144

non-IgE food reactions (nonallergic food hypersensitivities), 252, 261–262

non-immunologic drug reactions

  drug idiosyncrasy, 279–280, 284

  drug intolerances, 280, 284

nonnative plants, 88

non-specific reactivity, 38

nonsteroidal anti-inflammatory drugs (NSAIDs), 112, 232, 283, 285

nose and nasal health, 114–131. *See also* allergic rhinitis; otitis media; rhinitis; sinusitis

Not One More Life (NOML), 143

NRL (natural rubber latex), 214

NSAIDs (nonsteroidal anti-inflammatory drugs), 112, 232, 283, 285

O

OAS (oral allergy syndrome), 78–79, 257, 308

occupational allergic rhinitis, 64–65, 69

occupational asthma, 144

Occupational Safety and Health Administration (OSHA), 214

oily resin (oleoresin), 223. *See also* poison plants

OIT (oral immunotherapy), 77, 273–274

oleoresin (oily resin), 223. *See also* poison plants

olopatadine (Patanol; Pataday OTC), 62, 112

olopatadine and mometasone (Ryaltis), 108

olopatadine hydrochloride, 100–101

omalizumab (Xolair), 246, 275

OME (otitis media with effusion), 126, 129–130, 164

OMIT (oral mucosal immunotherapy), 77, 274

open challenges, 271

Opticrom (cromolyn sodium), 109, 112

Optivar Rx (azelastine), 62

oral allergy syndrome (OAS), 78–79, 257, 308

oral antibiotics

  contact dermatitis, 227

  urticaria and angioedema, 247

About the Authors

William E. Berger, MD, MBA, received his medical degree from the University of Cincinnati College of Medicine in 1973. He then completed an internship and residency program in pediatrics at the UCLA Medical Center in 1976. Dr. Berger pursued additional training at the National Jewish Hospital and Research Center where he served as a Fellow in Allergy and Immunology from 1976 to 1978. Board Certified in both pediatrics and allergy and immunology, Dr. Berger founded the Allergy and Asthma Associates of Southern California Medical Group in 1981 in Mission Viejo, Calif., where he practiced both adult and pediatric allergy.

In 1995, Dr. Berger established the Southern California Research Center, focusing on respiratory and allergy clinical research projects. To further his educational goals, in 1997, Dr. Berger received his master's degree in business administration from the Graduate School of Management of the University of California, Irvine. He held dual appointments as clinical professor at the College of Medicine, Department of Pediatrics, Division of Allergy and Immunology, and adjunct professor of Health Care Management in the Graduate School of Management at the University of California, Irvine.

Dr. Berger has served as president of the Orange County and California Societies of Allergy, Asthma, and Immunology. He has also been a member of the Joint Task Force on Practice Parameters, chairman of the Managed Care Committee of the American College of Allergy, Asthma & Immunology, and chairman of the Mission Hospital Institutional Review Board. Dr. Berger is a past president of the American College of Allergy, Asthma & Immunology, a professional organization that represents more than 6,000 allergy and asthma specialists throughout the United States and from many foreign countries. A former television medical correspondent for the Orange County Newschannel, Dr. Berger is the author of many academic papers and lay press articles in the field of allergy, asthma and immunology, including the recently published book *Asthma For Dummies*.

Dr. Berger presently serves as Medical Director and National Spokesperson for the Allergy & Asthma Network (AAN), a patient advocacy organization whose goal is "to improve quality of life and achieve equitable and health outcomes for adults and children living with these chronic conditions, especially those in underserved communities." AAN works with "national and local partners to train healthcare professionals and host events and screenings that reach people directly in their communities."

Nicole Faris, MS, holds a BS in Nutritional Sciences and a MS in Food Science & Technology from University College Cork (UCC), Ireland where she graduated with honors in 2001. Her diverse career spans over two decades, encompassing academia, industry, clinical research, patient advocacy, and scientific consulting. Over the course of her career, Nicole spent 15 years at a leading Fortune

500 company in Europe, assuming increasingly senior roles in medical affairs, scientific communications, and clinical research, gaining a strong foundation in immunology and allergy. During her tenure in industry, Nicole's expanding interest in allergies led her to pursue a dedicated allergy course for healthcare professionals in Southampton UK, where she engaged with, and was mentored, by the leading thought-leaders in the field.

In 2015, Nicole relocated with her family to the United States and established her own health consulting firm. In 2019, Nicole was afforded an invaluable opportunity to join a world-renowned allergy and immunology team based in Colorado, where she gained direct experience in clinical trial oversight and patient care, while working as a senior research supervisor.

More recently, she served as senior director at the largest food allergy research nonprofit in the United States. Collaborating closely with several global pharmaceutical companies, Nicole gained a wealth of expertise in drug development pathways, including the planning, execution, and oversight of clinical trials and patient advocacy. In her most recent career endeavor, Nicole returned to consulting, supporting small to medium-size enterprises in strategic planning, medical writing, and medical conference execution.

As a lifelong food allergy sufferer, Nicole is passionate about effective allergy care for patients and their families. This passion inspired a unique collaboration with the eminent Dr. Berger on this important book, and she is most grateful for the opportunity.

Dedication

Dr. Berger: This book is dedicated to my wife Charlette, my son Michael, my daughter Johanna, and my grandchildren Tyler, Shane, Nevada, and Brenna, for their loving encouragement and their inspiring confidence that I would actually get all the writing done on time.

Nicole: This book is dedicated to my husband Ryan, my daughter Lilia, and my father Eddie for your unwavering support and encouragement and your patience and faith in me as a new author. A heartfelt thanks for inspiring me to get this book over the finish line, I couldn't have done it without you.

Authors' Acknowledgments

It's hard to believe that it's been almost 20 years since *Allergies For Dummies* was published in 2006. During that time, great strides in the diagnosis and treatment of allergic disorders have occurred, which are now included in *Allergy For Dummies*.

We first want to thank acquisitions editor Elizabeth Stilwell, whose foresight and vision generated this publication and made this updated book possible. Our project editor, Chad Sievers kept us on track throughout the writing process and his guidance was greatly appreciated by everyone involved.

This book couldn't have been accomplished without the incredible direction of our indefatigable senior research editor, Carl Byron, whose guidance and perseverance kept us focused and productive and most importantly, who responded to all our texts, emails, and phone calls.

We also want to express our deep-felt appreciation to Phil Lieberman, MD, who acted as technical editor on this new update. The invaluable insights from his outstanding years of experience in the field of Allergy and Immunology can't be overstated, and we're greatly appreciative of his assistance and support.

Most of all, we'd like to thank all the patients with allergy and asthma conditions who have shared their stories with us and have provided their unique perspective and feedback to help develop a book that addresses their needs. We hope that *Allergy For Dummies* will be a significant additional resource to help these patients get the care they need and deserve, enabling them to lead happy, healthy, and productive lives.

Publisher's Acknowledgments

Acquisition Editor: Elizabeth Stilwell

Project Manager and Copy Editor: Chad R. Sievers

Technical Editor: Phil Lieberman, MD

Production Editor: Saikarthick Kumarasamy

Cover Image: © Volodymyr TVERDOKHLIB/ Shutterstock.com

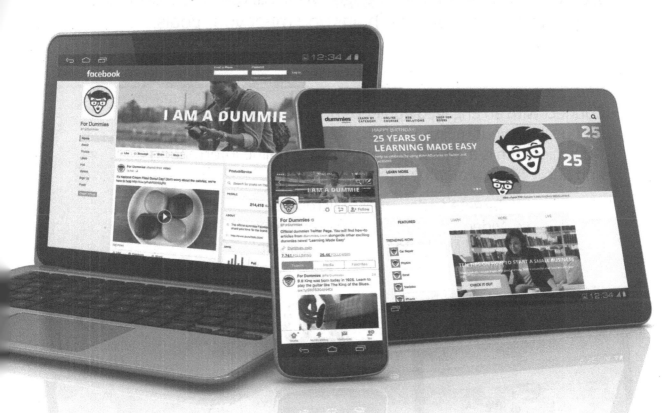
  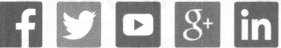

Leverage the power

Dummies is the global leader in the reference category and one of the most trusted and highly regarded brands in the world. No longer just focused on books, customers now have access to the dummies content they need in the format they want. Together we'll craft a solution that engages your customers, stands out from the competition, and helps you meet your goals.

Advertising & Sponsorships

Connect with an engaged audience on a powerful multimedia site, and position your message alongside expert how-to content. Dummies.com is a one-stop shop for free, online information and know-how curated by a team of experts.

- Targeted ads
- Video
- Email Marketing
- Microsites
- Sweepstakes sponsorship

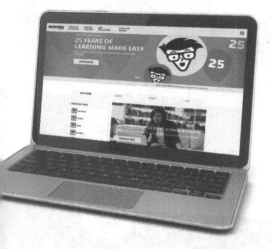

20 MILLION PAGE VIEWS EVERY SINGLE MONTH

15 MILLION UNIQUE VISITORS PER MONTH

43% OF ALL VISITORS ACCESS THE SITE VIA THEIR MOBILE DEVICES

700,000 NEWSLETTER SUBSCRIPTIONS TO THE INBOXES OF

300,000 UNIQUE INDIVIDUALS EVERY WEEK

# of dummies

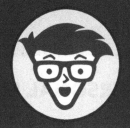

Custom Publishing

Reach a global audience in any language by creating a solution that will differentiate you from competitors, amplify your message, and encourage customers to make a buying decision.

- Apps
- Books
- eBooks
- Video
- Audio
- Webinars

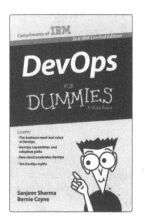 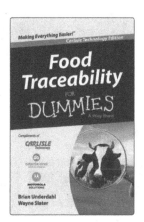 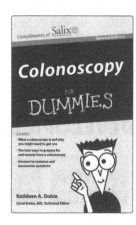 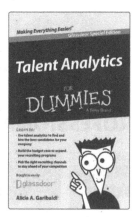

Brand Licensing & Content

Leverage the strength of the world's most popular reference brand to reach new audiences and channels of distribution.

For more information, visit dummies.com/biz

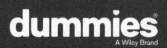

PERSONAL ENRICHMENT

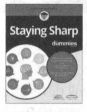
Staying Sharp
9781119187790
USA $26.00
CAN $31.99
UK £19.99

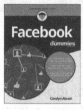
Facebook
9781119179030
USA $21.99
CAN $25.99
UK £16.99

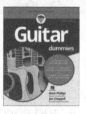
Guitar
9781119293354
USA $24.99
CAN $29.99
UK £17.99

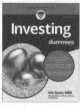
Investing
9781119293347
USA $22.99
CAN $27.99
UK £16.99

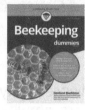
Beekeeping
9781119310068
USA $22.99
CAN $27.99
UK £16.99

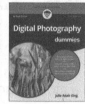
Digital Photography
9781119235606
USA $24.99
CAN $29.99
UK £17.99

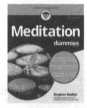
Meditation
9781119251163
USA $24.99
CAN $29.99
UK £17.99

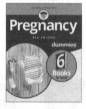
Pregnancy
9781119235491
USA $26.99
CAN $31.99
UK £19.99

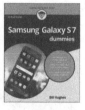
Samsung Galaxy S7
9781119279952
USA $24.99
CAN $29.99
UK £17.99

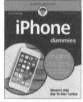
iPhone
9781119283133
USA $24.99
CAN $29.99
UK £17.99

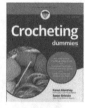
Crocheting
9781119287117
USA $24.99
CAN $29.99
UK £16.99

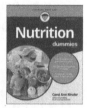
Nutrition
9781119130246
USA $22.99
CAN $27.99
UK £16.99

PROFESSIONAL DEVELOPMENT

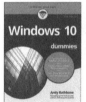
Windows 10
9781119311041
USA $24.99
CAN $29.99
UK £17.99

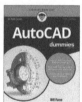
AutoCAD
9781119255796
USA $39.99
CAN $47.99
UK £27.99

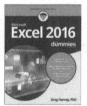
Excel 2016
9781119293439
USA $26.99
CAN $31.99
UK £19.99

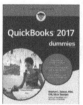
QuickBooks 2017
9781119281467
USA $26.99
CAN $31.99
UK £19.99

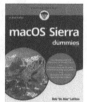
macOS Sierra
9781119280651
USA $29.99
CAN $35.99
UK £21.99

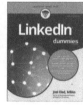
LinkedIn
9781119251132
USA $24.99
CAN $29.99
UK £17.99

Windows 10 All-in-One
9781119310563
USA $34.00
CAN $41.99
UK £24.99

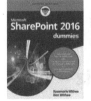
SharePoint 2016
9781119181705
USA $29.99
CAN $35.99
UK £21.99

Fundamental Analysis
9781119263593
USA $26.99
CAN $31.99
UK £19.99

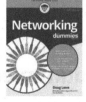
Networking
9781119257769
USA $29.99
CAN $35.99
UK £21.99

Office 2016
9781119293477
USA $26.99
CAN $31.99
UK £19.99

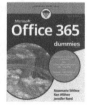
Office 365
9781119265313
USA $24.99
CAN $29.99
UK £17.99

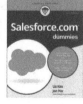
Salesforce.com
9781119239314
USA $29.99
CAN $35.99
UK £21.99

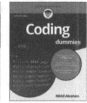
Coding
9781119293323
USA $29.99
CAN $35.99
UK £21.99

dummies.com

dummies
A Wiley Brand